Wake Up With a New Smile

Wake Up With a New Smile

The Smart Consumer's Guide to
DENTISTRY

Dr. Joseph G. Marcius, DDS
with Dr. Charles W. Martin, DDS

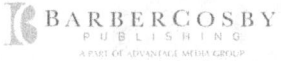
BARBERCOSBY
PUBLISHING
A PART OF ADVANCE MEDIA GROUP

Published by BarberCosby, Charleston, South Carolina.
Member of Advantage Media Group.

BARBERCOSBY is a registered trademark and the BarbyCosby colophon is a trademark of Advantage Media Group, Inc.
Printed in the United States of America.

ISBN: 978-1-59932-191-2
LCCN: 2011905968

This publication is designed to provide accurate and authoritative information in regard to the subject matter covered. It is sold with the understanding that the publisher is not engaged in rendering legal, accounting, or other professional services. If legal advice or other expert assistance is required, the services of a competent professional person should be sought.

Most Advantage Media Group titles are available at special quantity discounts for bulk purchases for sales promotions, premiums, fundraising, and educational use. Special versions or book excerpts can also be created to fit specific needs.
For more information, please write: Special Markets, Advantage Media Group, P.O. Box 272, Charleston, SC 29402 or call 1.866.775.1696.

Visit us online at **barbercosby**.com

Contact Us:

Joseph G. Marcius, DDS
Chapel Hill Dental Care
1690 Brittain Road
Akron, Ohio 44310
Office: 330-633-711
Fax: 330-633-8837
DrJoeMarcius@earthlink.net

Contents

Preface:

Why do we need a new book on dentistry? First, because dentistry has changed. A lot. And if you have the same opinion of dentistry as you've always had, that view should change as well. Because doing so can save your teeth, and as you'll learn, your health.

Not only that, it can also help save you time and money. It can help you make wise choices that could improve your life.

This book can help you or a loved one make a wise choice about dental care. Too often we see people make choices about their dentistry for the wrong reasons.

This book can be a counsel for you on choosing the right treatments and about what makes good common sense for you. Once you know all the effects that your teeth have on you, I think it's going to change the way you think about your teeth and oral health and your overall being.

It can teach you what you need to know to be a smart consumer, to make smart choices. You know, the joint health community has not educated people about their teeth, and it's still not happening despite the work of the Surgeon General's Report on Oral Health 2000.

 Visit www.surgeongeneral.gov/library/oralhealth for more information.

Hopefully, reading this book can make a meaningful difference in your life. What value do teeth provide? Well, number one, they improve how you look. Your beauty or good looks is directly affected by your teeth. How you look does matter. How people treat you is directly related to how you look, whether we like it or not. This is particularly true early on in any new relationship. Your looks have a big effect on the person you're getting to know. So it has a direct effect on relationships.

We know from studies, this one from the American Dental Association published in 2007, that 81% of people consider your smile the most dominant feature of your facial appearance. Wow! There are billions spent on skin care; there are more billions spent on everything else you can think of under the sun, moon and stars related to appearance that have nothing to do with your smile.

Your smile has a direct effect on how people perceive you; your likability, your desirability. Speaking of desirability, what about the effect on romance? Often we see patients come in our office that have had a recent divorce. They're down and have decided they need to spruce themselves up and have a smile makeover. Get the look they've always wanted. You know, from the standpoint of romance, a gorgeous smile makes a big difference in how attractive and desirable you are.

Your teeth have a big effect on your comfort. Unfortunately, too many people ignore their teeth until there's a problem, until there's true discomfort. This discomfort can be mild at first and then become excruciating pain. We know that your teeth affect your business and professional life. If your job involves working with other people, you have to be able to positively influence them just to get along in the work place. If your work has to do with persuading and moving them to your way of thinking, a good-looking smile is a requirement. In today's highly competitive workplace you need every edge possible.

This book just might move you to take better care of your teeth, which in turn, could vastly improve, or even save, your life. Most people probably know very little about their teeth and how it affects their health, and more importantly – neither do most people in the health care industry. So along with general information about modern dentistry and how to make choices about it, this book will shed light on the interdependence of oral health and overall health.

Doctors industry-wide are beginning to understand that those people who get their teeth fixed and keep them healthy live longer, better quality lives. Some estimate this increase in longevity at ten years!

Healthy teeth help you function normally, help you effectively chew the foods you like to eat. They enable you to speak, smile, and get along in life. And they powerfully and directly affect your health. We know that your oral health has a direct relationship to the rest of your body. It affects your cardiovascular system; it affects arthritis, heart disease, stroke, diabetes.

We're finding that the inflammation caused by the infections in your mouth, even the kind that doesn't hurt and remains invisible, affects your body's ability to handle stress in general.

Research is now pointing to inflammation as a probable cause of Alzheimer's Disease. This horrible, debilitating condition chokes the life out of its victims and worsens the lives of caregivers, usually the family members who love them. Chronic, often symptom-less dental infections that so many older people have can and do cause inflammation throughout the body. Many dental problems that numerous people have deemed "innocent" and "no big deal" could be a very big deal in what are supposed to be the golden years of life. Who wants to become a burden to their loved ones? More research is needed, but we already know that infections in the mouth can seep into the body from neglected and painless dental disease. Why put your future at risk unnecessarily?

You Will Need Your Teeth Longer

Longevity is increasing. Today, we know that half of those who are age 60 or older are going to live to be in their nineties. We've made sweeping changes in how long people live. At the time that social security was implemented, the average life span was 47 years! So it was very easy to provide a system that gave retirement benefits at age 65.

Today, we're tipping out over 80 on average and it's climbing. With the Human Genome Project and the advances in nanotechnology, we expect that life spans are going to be over 100 years in the not so distant future. How far in the future is anyone's guess, but like everything else, we expect the pace of longevity and how long people live to accelerate as we know more about health and how it affects you.

One of the big lessons of this book is how to keep your teeth for your lifetime, even to age 100! We want readers to not only add years to their life, but life to their years.

When I ask my patients what is the one thing that helps keep them coming back? They say, "I want to keep my teeth!" Many times they have a parent who has lost their teeth and seen, first hand, the misery that comes with tooth loss.

In these pages we'll address, head-on, the common anxiety and fear so many patients experience - so you can get the care you need comfortably. Frankly, we're dismayed and saddened when we hear of patients who don't come in because they're fearful. We'll show you how modern dentistry can help you to conquer that fear, and why today those fears have in large-part, become baseless.

We're going to talk about what works and what doesn't work in treatment.

Unfortunately, much of the care that people ask for isn't long-lasting. Part of our diagnosis and treatment process is concentrating on care that will endure, and be the most beneficial for the longest time.

We'll look into the latest advanced treatments and their advantages and disadvantages. And we'll talk about the "expedient" procedures to avoid.

Why? Because sometimes such expedient dentistry actually sets you up for bigger, more expensive problems in the future. Sadly, we see it every day.

We'll help you see dentistry from the perspective of a dentist who is treating you.

We're going to talk about how much you should expect to pay for different levels of health care. This is important, so I'll repeat that again. We're going to talk about how much you should expect to pay for different levels of dental care. There is a difference and you need to know about it.

You can read this book in one of several different ways. You can turn to the chapter that applies to you right now, or you can turn to the beginning and read it cover to cover. It doesn't matter. What we want for you is that this book has application to your life, answers your questions and increases your knowledge so you can be a smart dental consumer.

You'll be able to access further information on the topics we cover on the Web. Look for this special icon to find these links throughout the book.

At the end of the book, you'll find a chapter about me, and about how I became a dentist. I'll tell you about my current practice and provide contact information and special certificates for readers. So, if you would like to find us or doctors like us, you can.

The stories of patients told herein are composite stories of real patients. We have altered names and put these together to help you understand dental care and its benefits in a new way. The reality is that the new, more modern dentist can be a real source of greater health, a better quality of life and a longer one. The power they wield can be regenerative, even transformative to a whole new, better level of living.

A beautiful smile. Healthy teeth for life. Better total health. The look that speaks and tells untold volumes. A great smile says a lot about how you think about yourself. And it give you that first edge when dealing with people from anywhere. Our society assigns attributes to more attractive people – and your smile is the major component of that.

Attractive people are considered to be smarter, more desirable, friendlier, and "better". Better in so many ways. And your smile is the centerfold of it all.

Perhaps you have witnessed firsthand the effects a power smile has had on a new acquaintance, a close friend or even a dear relative. Perhaps the effect it has had on you. It is not a pretty picture. And it doesn't have to be that way any longer.

It is true that you no long have to suffer with smile and teeth disabilities. So much is possible today that wasn't before.

Life altering dental care, described here, happens everyday.

Through these stories, you will learn to better appreciate the importance of healthy teeth and a beautiful smile.

When you are ready to learn even more about your situation, then it is as simple as making a phone call to get you on the path to a great smile, better health and teeth for a lifetime.

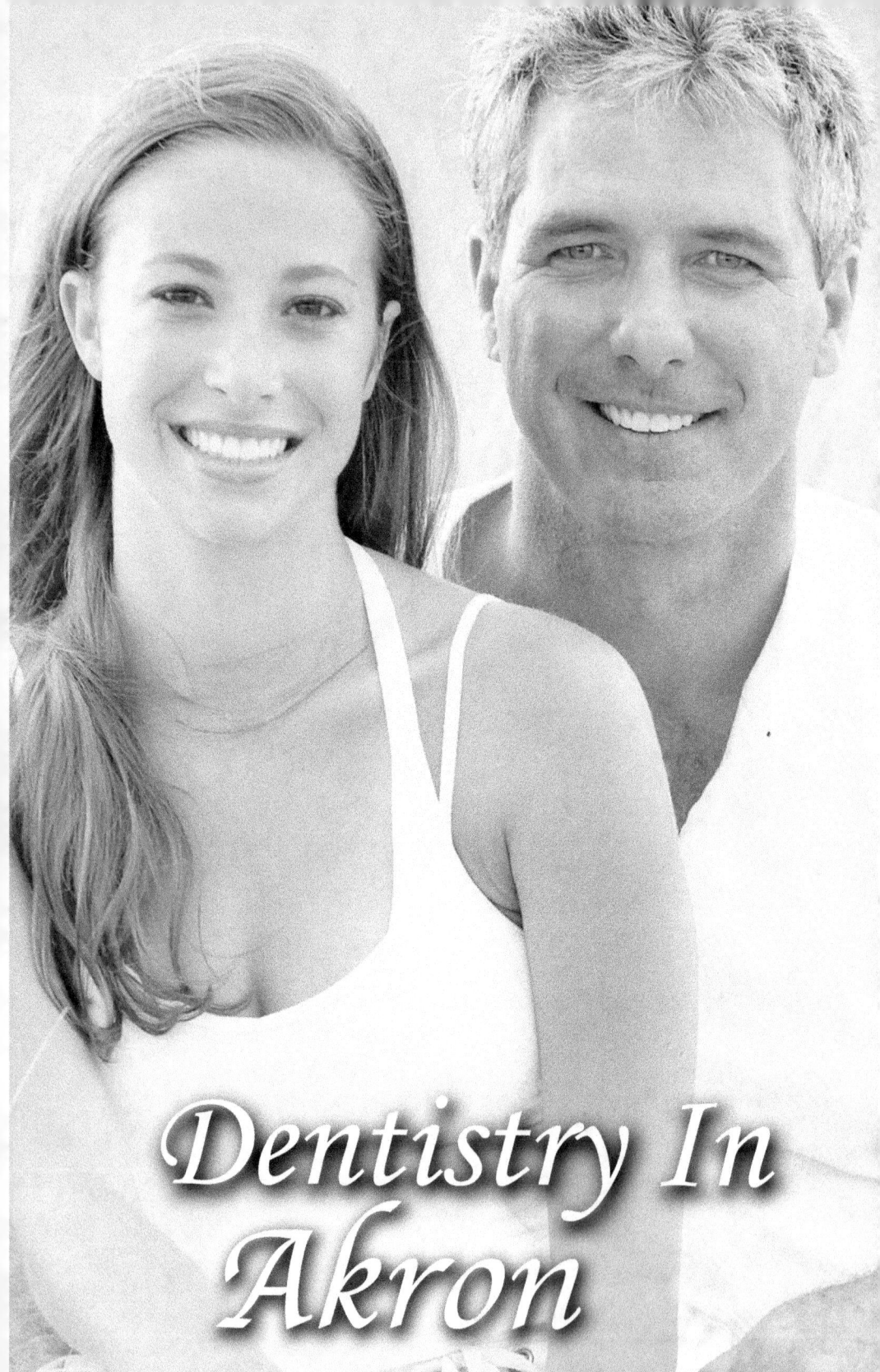

Dentistry In Akron

CHAPTER 1
Dentistry In Akron
by Dr. Joseph G. Marcius

A criminal prosecutor who swims with sharks, Sarah finds adventure in things most people fear. She'll scuba dive off the Pacific coast and fight crime in the courtroom—but when it comes to the dentist, Sarah would rather swim with the Hammerheads.

Sarah is like many patients who visit my office. They cringe at the hum of dental drills and wince at the scraping of chisel against teeth. They feel nauseous, on-edge and sleep-deprived before an appointment. Their anxiety is so crippling that they avoid the dentist at all costs, a risk to their oral health and physical well-being.

I believe no patient should be deprived treatment due to fear. I want you to know that you have options when choosing your dentist, that if you have been written off as hopeless or labeled as "untreatable" due to anxiety or other medical complications, you no longer have to settle for compromised care.

So what makes my approach different? Because I know what it's like to be afraid.

I used to dread dental appointments. Teeth cleanings, oral exams—you name it. I would fixate on the frosted waiting room window separating me from the receptionist, hoping against hope she would not call my name next.

But you won't experience that at my office. Imagine a dental facility without the notorious sliding glass front desk window or dimly lit examination rooms. What if instead you walked into an office with soothing music and sunlight streaming in—a place that felt a little more like home? How would that change your perception of dentistry?

From making the first appointment to your in-office consultation, my staff and I will listen to your concerns and shape an individualized treatment plan to meet your needs. After more than 18 years of practicing intravenous (IV) sedation—a means of providing dental care while the patient appears to sleep—I continue to seek the best methods for treating high-anxiety individuals. Patients who come to my practice know this is not the dental office they have come to fear. And this is the experience I want for you.

When I graduated from Case Western Reserve University School of Dental Medicine, dentistry was primarily concerned with the function of teeth. Unappealing dentures were used to solve any problem with unhealthy teeth. Basic chewing ability trumped aesthetic appeal, and few professionals focused on how a beautiful smile can enhance a person's quality of life.

Complex care dentistry is needed in today's society where big pearly whites are considered essential to job placement, sex appeal and self-confidence. But the old-school mentality of high-patient turnover and 15 minute check-ups cannot bring the results most patients expect. For this reason, I have invested thousands of hours into continuing education, attending seminars, conferences and courses to learn the most current techniques dentistry has to offer.

Many of my colleagues in the Akron, Ohio area now refer their most anxious or medically compromised patients to my practice. I treat those who fear needles and experience gag reflex or who have conditions such as Turrets, Parkinson's and Down's syndrome. Patients who have intolerance to local anesthesia often seek my care.

Whether or not you are like these patients, you can experience the benefits of a smile makeover at my office. I start by sculpting your temporaries, the teeth worn prior to completing the porcelain reconstruction of your smile. Using a photo of you as a reference tool, I design the teeth to fit the contour of your mouth and the shape of your face, keeping in mind proportionality and balance. You will then have the opportunity to see the temporaries in place, where we can make the adjustments that you want before creating the final product: your new smile.

We end your experience with a complementary professional portrait session at my photography studio right here in the office. Patients who have not smiled in years often find it liberating to dress up and finally show off their teeth. This is my way of showing that I care and that I love what I do.

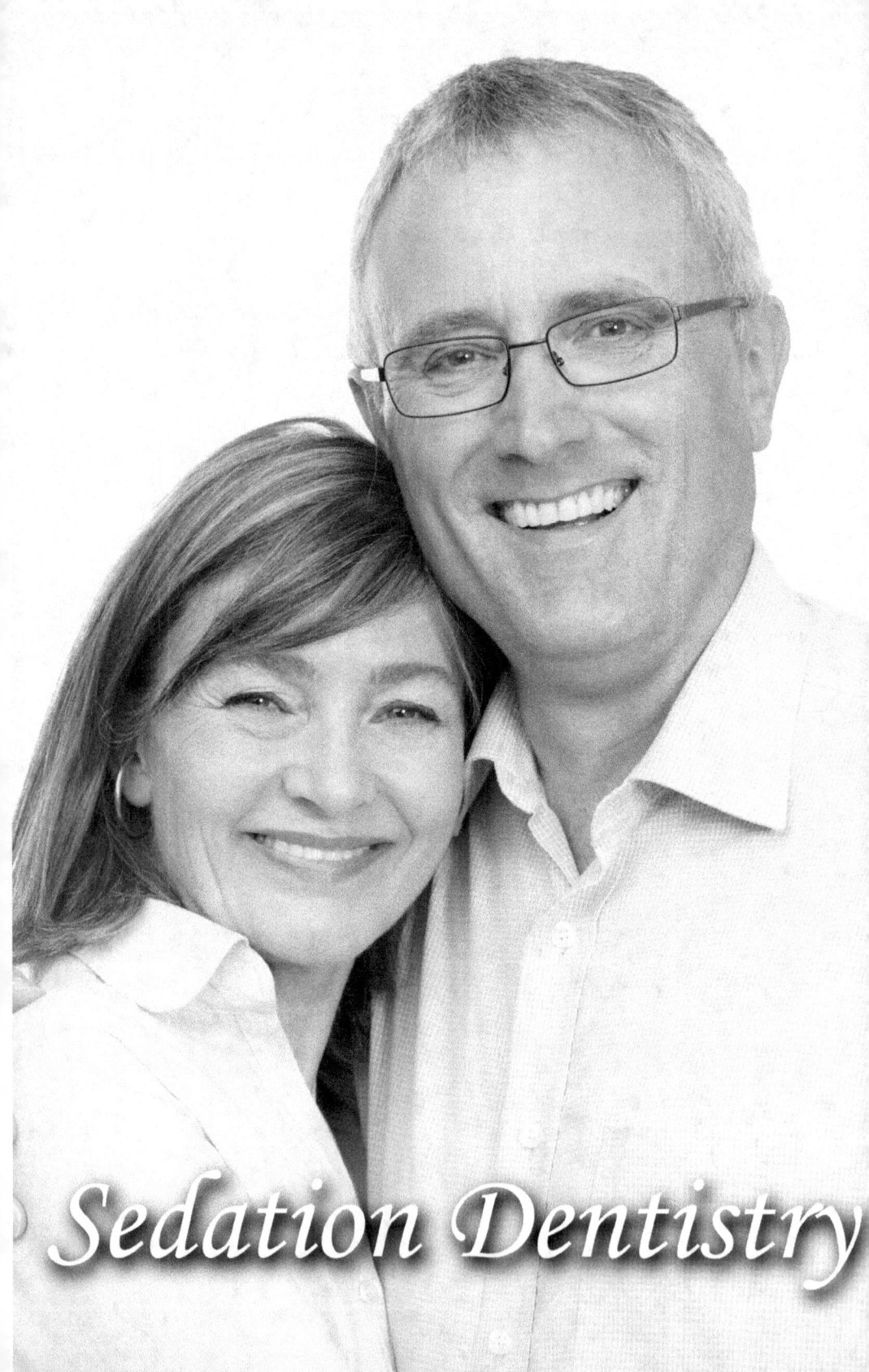

Sedation Dentistry

CHAPTER 2
Sedation Dentistry

Do you think there's no such thing as a comfortable, relaxing dental visit?

Maybe your dentist has been holding out on you. If you've got pain or fear, no worries, sedation is here.

Did you know that 75% of all Americans experience feelings of anxiety about going to the dentist? In fact, some 30 million Americans are deathly afraid of going to the dentist.

So, if you have a fear or an anxiety, you're not alone.

I realize that as an intelligent knowledgeable person, you already understand the importance of healthy gums and teeth. And you know how they enhance your good looks, give you a more youthful appearance, keep you pain-free, as well as promote overall good health.

I also know that doesn't amount to a hill of beans when queasiness and terror seize your body at the thought of visiting a dentist. It doesn't have to be that way.

Good dentists realize that whether your aversion of the dentist comes from hearing one too many horror stories or from a traumatic experience of your own, that the fear is real. No amount of wishing is going to make it go away.

A good dentist understands that just because you haven't seen the dentist in years doesn't mean that you don't care about your health or that you're too cheap or that you have no sense of personal hygiene. You do care. You would spend the money if you could.

The problem is that paralyzing fear that you can't seem to shake.

We can help.

We understand that it's not rational thinking keeping you out of our offices. It's irrational emotion that freezes you.

The good news! With conscious sedation dentistry, you have a new way to get the care that you desperately need without the pain, fear or unpleasantness you've always expected.

And despite what you may have been told or heard in the past, there is a pleasant, safe, easy way for you to stop suffering from the horrible hidden costs in not getting proper dental care.

You no longer have to be embarrassed by your teeth. You no longer have to hide your grin, use phony smile tricks or live in pain.

Sedation dentistry helps you reclaim your health and your good looks with comfort and relaxation.

It can help you completely relax at your dental appointments. It may sound impossible. But with this technique you can lightly "snooze" right through your dental appointment. In most cases, patients don't actually fall asleep, but they do experience a deep feeling of calm and peace.

When combined with careful application of a numbing agent to any sensitive areas, patients experience a virtually pain-free relaxing session for their dental care.

So, who is sedation dentistry for? It's for those who want the dental care they need without the pain and fear they've come to expect.

It's useful if you…

- Have fears that make you delay or avoid proper dental care.

- Have had a bad experience with dentists in the past.

- Have a strong gag reflex.

- Suffer acute or chronic jaw soreness.

- Dislike the sights, sounds and smells associated with a dental office.

- Have trouble getting numb.

- Need a lot of work to be done but don't have time for several appointments.

- You're embarrassed about the condition of your teeth and want to take action.

- Hate the sight of needles

- Have physical limitations such as back or neck problems.

So, what does sedation feel like? Mostly, like a catnap. You're not unconscious, but you're pleasantly "dozing" as though in a half waking, half dream state.

Most patients report feeling just unaware enough to become relaxed. And when it's all over, you feel refreshed with little or no memory of the treatment performed.

There are two different methods for sedation that I use, Oral Sedation and Intravenous Sedation. Let's talk about oral sedation first.

What's it like? First you'll receive a small pill, usually a mild sedative to take the night before your appointment. This will help you sleep through the night so you feel relaxed and stress free and get a good night's sleep.

Then, about a half an hour before your appointment the next morning, you take another pill to soothe your nerves and calm your mind.

Now, let's talk about Intravenous Sedation. This technique is used for patients when oral sedation does not provide the level of sedation needed for the appointment. Multiple doses of the drug can be given,

What Are the Hidden Costs of Suffering With Bad Teeth?

- Romances snuffed out because of chipped, jumbled, broken or missing teeth that create an unpleasant smile, that repel that certain someone you want noticing you.

- Tender or sensitive, uncomfortable teeth.

- A loss of the ability to enjoy your favorite foods.

- Dreading every social or outing event because people may notice and be turned off by your smile.

- Worsening nutrition and health.

- Outright pain every time you bite down.

- Having your children or grandchildren comment or even make fun of your teeth.

- Lessened self-confidence.

- Losing a promotion that could have been yours.

- The ever increasing unsightly gaps between your teeth that worsen as you grow older.

- Even threats to your health.

if needed, throughout the appointment. This is often necessary for those patients already taking anti-anxiety medications, patients with special needs (Alzheimer's, Turrettes,MS,etc.), and people requiring long appointments. Sometimes the oral sedation may stop working on some people on long appointments before the procedure is completed.

IV Sedation can even be done even if you are afraid of needles. We can give you Nitrous Oxide gas (laughing gas) first to help relax you. Once you are relaxed and comfortable in the dental chair, we will cover you with a warm blanket. You can bring your headphones to listen to your own music. Then, an anesthetic cream can be placed on your arm. This numbs the area where the IV will be placed, making the process more comfortable for you. You are then given the sedative drug. Your dental care is done for you without you being aware. Then, before you know it, you are leaving out the door as if it never happened.

What happens after the appointment? You still may feel a bit sleepy. That's why I encourage you to take it easy and rest comfortably until a friend or family member picks you up.

We don't want you to drive and will probably prefer that you rest for the remainder of the day.

You are encouraged to eat and drink as you desire. And by the next morning, everything should be back to a normal routine.

Sedation is very safe. Throughout your entire appointment you'll be carefully monitored.

Of course, we're going to make sure that you're doing well during your sedated state.

Are there side effects? Well, patients often report little or no memory of their treatment experience. Frequently patients will call to say they were amazed they don't remember anything much about the dental care.

And when asked to look in the mirror, patients often gasp and shed tears of joy when they realize how improved their teeth and smiles are. And the fact they don't remember much is one of their favorite side effects.

Another positive side effect is reduced soreness that's a result of being so relaxed during the process. Some may also get a dry mouth because sedatives can decrease salivary flow. And about 3% of patients have some hiccups.

So, should you have sedation dentistry?

If you have fears that are preventing you from getting the care you need, then, yes.

Not long ago we had a patient named Simon. Simon was a big guy, weighing probably between 280 and 300 pounds. He was 6 '4". But he was still frightened of the dentist.

When he sat down he looked a little bit more than nervous. In fact, he was shaking. Simon had put off a lot of dentistry. But he also knew he had to get something done. So, he literally forced himself to come into the office.

When we started talking about using sedation as an alternative to help him get through his appointment, he was elated. Even before he stopped shaking, he said, "Okay. This sounds good."

We had to do a lot of work on Simon. But surprisingly, after a couple of appointments using sedation, Simon no longer wanted it.

He said, "You know doc, I've gotten comfortable enough I don't need that anymore." Today Simon is smiling largely, happily and no longer needs sedation when he comes to see us.

This is true of a lot of our sedation patients.

Peter's Story

Peter's wife pulled me aside. She told me, "What you did has been magical in our lives. You know, I was the skeptic. I was the one who didn't want him to have this work done. I was the one who felt like it was going to be too much money and we couldn't afford it. Now Peter is sooo much better. He has more energy. He plays with the kids. He has a brighter mood. He used to come home always disturbed and exhausted at the end of the day and he's not like that anymore. He likes people. We go out with our friends more; and he's a whole lot nicer to me. Now is it all because you fixed his smile? I'm not sure, but boy, is it better now. It has been so worth it."

I thanked her for her words. Peter had huge problems – serious, major-major ones. We have come to expect little life miracles with our patients like Peter after we complete our smile make-overs. Many times it's going to become a transformational event that changes the individual physically. That was certainly true for Peter. His transformation at the physical level led to multiple changes in many other dimensions of his life. Peter told me that he had gotten two promotions in the past two years and a 40% salary increase. I said, "To what do you attribute that, Peter?" He says, "I'm a different person now. I'm smiling at people more and they are smiling back at me. Before I was a bit of a grump, and I didn't smile at people. My boss got promoted and had to leave. He recommended me for his position. I took it. Now I'm being promoted again and I'm going to have a five state region to deal work with. And as you guess my pay went up again, so I'm pleased as punch. Thank you Dr. for all you've done."

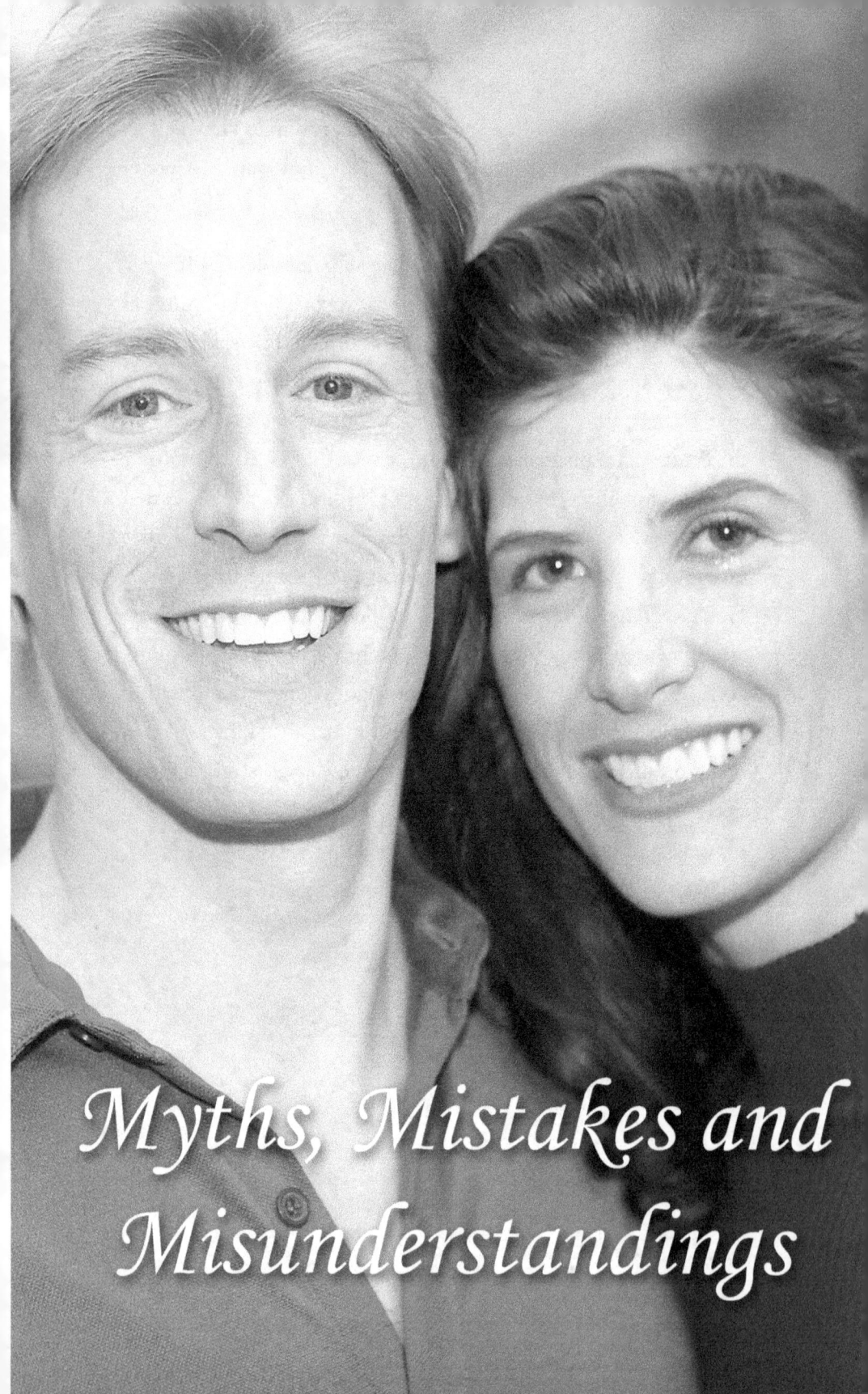

Myths, Mistakes and
Misunderstandings

CHAPTER 3
Myths, Mistakes and Misunderstandings:
It's What People Don't Know That Gets Them In Trouble

There are a lot of myths about dental care, teeth, dentists and oral health. The mistakes that people make with their teeth are needless; if they really understood the decisions they were making far fewer mistakes would be made. The purpose of this section is to set the record straight, prevent the mistakes and to dispel the myths and misunderstandings that get people in trouble with their teeth.

( ) Myth 1: "A dentist is a dentist is a dentist."

Nothing could be further from the truth.

Think of it this way: if you were hiring an attorney to buy a house, you would hire a real estate attorney. If you were going to a courtroom, you would hire a litigator. If you're going to hire an architect to build a house, you'd hire a very different architect than the one paid to develop a whole city.

Likewise, it's important for you to understand just what type of dentist you need. For many, a regular family dentist is the right answer. For others, that's not nearly enough. The more serious your dental needs are, the more experience, training, talent, skill, and judgment you need. One reason for this book is to help you know the difference.

( ) Myth 2 : "My regular dentist can handle everything."

Most often, this isn't the case. In fact, it's dangerous to assume that your dentist knows everything that you need him to know. Be skeptical, and understand that sometimes you need to find the dentist who has more care, skill and training. The gap between dentists – in skill, knowledge, and training – is greater than it has ever been.

( ) Myth 3: "When they get bad, just take them out."

Boy, if this were only the right solution, we would love it! Removing the offending tooth does make sense in a way: it gets rid of the pain. But every time you remove a tooth there is a whole series of chain reactions that occur: your other teeth move. The gap or space created causes additional stresses on other teeth, often resulting in an impaired chewing function, gum disease and loss of still more teeth.

If simply yanking teeth were the end-all solution, people would just take all their teeth out and get dentures. In fact, for a time in certain countries, including Canada, this was thought to be the ultimate wedding gift: To remove all the teeth and give the wedding couple dentures. Seriously. That way they would always avoid dental problems in the future. But we know that's not true. In fact, dentures are the equivalent of oral wigs, and most people are much more satisfied with wearing their own hair than with wearing a wig.

( ) Myth 4: "Dentures work just fine. My daddy had them, and he did just fine."

The truth is - some people can tolerate anything. We've seen people who don't wear dentures at all that manage to eat. And though it's an extreme exception, I've seen people who wear upper dentures with no lower denture. Again, this is a rare exception.

But what about normal dentures? How often does a person who has dentures "function normally?" One in ten at best. My guess is it's closer to one in fifteen. Unfortunately you won't know if you can tolerate dentures until you've lost all your teeth.

In the upcoming chapter on dental implants, I'll explain a lot more about the problems of dentures.

( ) Myth 5: "No one can see the back ones; it will be just fine to only fix the front."

If I just had a nickel for every time I've heard that one! However insane the sentiment seems, it does point out one thing: that people value the appearance of their smile. And indeed, a lot of times people can't see the back ones.

But there are serious problems with such logic. Your back teeth are made for chewing and grinding your food. The front teeth are made for viewing. If you try to chew with the teeth made for view, the teeth will break down. The back teeth are there for a reason. They give you the ability to chew and to function.

Think of your front teeth like a pair of scissors: they're good for incising, smiling, speaking, singing, and expressing yourself. But they aren't so good for chewing up a steak. It just doesn't work well. And in fact, just like a pair of scissors, when you try to chew with your front teeth, you wear out the edges, your teeth shorten, start to break down and break off. Not good.

( ) Myth 6: "My poorly aligned bite isn't that big a deal."

Actually, it may be a very big deal. We know that for some people, their bite being off causes them pain with chewing, pain to the jaw joints, pain in the neck, and chronic headaches. In fact, some estimate that over 75% of all headaches are muscle-contraction headaches that could be related to a poor bite.

If you think of your head as about a six-pound ball sitting on your spine, balanced by all the muscles in the neck and the face and the head, you realize that when one muscle or several muscles get into a bad place – a strained position – it can pull in such a way that all the other muscles are strained. And that muscle straining causes muscle contraction. Those contractions can cause headaches.

We often find that people whose bite is off will accommodate by changing their neck posture. And as soon as their neck posture changes, they start to have neck pain. This frequently occurs with computer users who sit in front of a monitor all day long.

Additionally, whenever you affect the spine, that effect ripples from the top to the bottom of the spine. Not only that, bite misalignment can cause you to break or crack teeth, or cause the dental work to wear prematurely, excessively or even fail. So, the bite being off can be a very big deal.

We know that a bad bite causes a lot of stress to the entire chewing mechanism, and this stress doesn't relieve itself easily. It takes time and a lot of relaxation. So I sometimes see people that are heavily medicated just to put up with their pain. It isn't necessary.

I've seen people whose bite is off who have accommodated for years and years and suddenly, because of their other stresses in life, they no longer have the "body energy" necessary to maintain themselves in spite of that bad bite, and things start to go downhill.

Often, and to my dismay, I hear: "This is the way God made me, so it must be okay." Well, it isn't okay. When you can't see, most get a set of glasses or contact lenses or have some type of surgery to correct things. If your hand isn't working correctly, almost anyone would seek therapy and sometimes surgery to get his hand functioning correctly. The "God made me this way" argument usually doesn't work out so well. Wouldn't you agree?

( ) Myth 7: "Dentists really aren't well trained anyway – at least not like real doctors."

All dentists have four years of undergraduate education, four years of dental school, and the good ones have myriad continuing education beyond that. Some have training well beyond the scope of what most average doctors receive.

Dentists ARE trained. And today we're actually helping to train the medical community to understand the connection between the mouth and the whole body. And together with our medical colleagues we're beginning to realize the impact of stress and bacterial infection from tooth decay and gum disease and its effect on your whole body.

( ) Myth 8: "My teeth don't really matter that much."

Wrong. Your teeth do matter. They matter at every level: Your looks, your health, your own self-concept, and how long you live. Keep reading and you'll never hold onto that myth again. Man is the only mammal that can live at all without its teeth. All other mammals die without their teeth. Do you think the loss of your teeth is innocuous? Think again.

( ) Myth 9: "My parents both lost their teeth, so my problems must be hereditary."

Just because your parents lost their teeth doesn't mean you will, too. Are some dental problems hereditary? Yes. How often is the heredity the reason that you have a dental problem? Very, very, seldom.

Only in a very small percentage of cases is heredity the reason that a patient loses his teeth. Just because Mom and Dad lost their teeth due to gum disease doesn't mean that you will. It's more likely they didn't care for their teeth, or didn't know how to. The purpose of this book is for you to know how to care for your teeth so you don't lose them.

( ) Myth 10: "Lose a tooth for every child."

I've heard this from many a mother. There is no evidence of any sort that supports the concept that for every baby that is born, you will lose a tooth. Yes, it is true that your body does go through physiologic changes during pregnancy. That's normal, but it doesn't mean you are destined to lose a tooth or even should.

◖◗ Myth 11: "My gums always bleed when I brush my teeth, so it must be normal."

Nope. When you brush your hair, do you expect your scalp to bleed? I think not. Bleeding gums are the first sign of inflammation, and inflammation is, today, considered a prime menace to your overall health. So no, bleeding gums are not normal. Just because it happens all the time doesn't make it normal.

We now know bleeding gums are caused by the inflammatory reaction to infections in your gums and around your teeth. And every infection, no matter where it occurs in the body, is a health threat that should be treated.

◖◗ Myth 12: "I drink sodas instead of coffee because they are better for me."

Please read carefully. Sodas contain acids that can easily eat through the enamel of the teeth. And the lighter-colored sodas actually have more acid. So if you're using sodas as a caffeine substitute for coffee, you are risking your teeth and your overall health.

In fact, when I see a patient come in as an adult or even as a teenager and I see a lot of decay, the first question I ask is, "Do you drink a lot of sodas?" because those soft drinks eat away at your teeth.

Often, in response, I hear, "Well, I really don't drink that many, I only sip on them." Well, sipping counts. Even when it's a diet drink, the acids work against you. Then, in a cruel chain of events, the substitute sweeteners in the diet drinks enable other sugars that come in contact with your teeth to create a rich environment for bacteria to explode in number and size, producing acids and enzymes that dissolve your teeth.

So don't substitute sodas for coffee. Not that I'm endorsing coffee. Whatever you drink, it's the sipping all day long without cleaning your teeth that creates a problem. If you're going to drink your coffee, drink it. If you're going to have your soda, drink it. But try to rinse with water afterwards. Rinsing this way helps stop decay problems before they start.

( ) Myth 13: "My diabetes has nothing to do with my dental health."

Fact is, if you're diabetic, you are 200% to 400% more likely to have gum disease. And, if you have dental problems, it makes your diabetes worse. And your diabetes makes your dental problems worse. It is a closed loop. Each affects the other.

We see that diabetes and dental health have a very, very strong relationship with one another. In fact, if you're diabetic or pre-diabetic, one of the best things you can do for yourself is get your teeth fixed and keep them that way.

Good dental health improves your ability to control your diabetes. Good diabetic control lessens your dental problems and makes it easier to keep that way. Most often those with diabetes should be seen every three to four months for maintenance therapy.

( ) Myth 14: "I go every six months, so I can't really have too many problems."

Well, that may be true and it may not be. We see individuals go every six months for regular care and have it work very well.

But beware. If you have untreated or undertreated problems in your mouth, maintenance visits every six months won't be enough. Incomplete care and untreated problems are a sort of "watchful waiting" that unnecessarily leads to worsening conditions, loss of teeth, more discomfort and more expense to treat.

We're going to talk about this more when we talk about gum disease, but for now understand that if you do not floss daily, you probably should go more often than every six months.

Rule number one is that you should probably use some type of device to help clean <u>between your teeth because as an adult about 85%</u> of all your problems occur between teeth where a toothbrush can't reach.

( ) Myth 15: "I only do what I have to do to get out of pain, but that's it."

Boy, that's a shame, because pain is only an indicator of a problem that's gotten so bad that it causes pain. Many dental problems don't cause pain at all until the problem is so bad that the offending tooth, gum needs significant treatment. Ouch. Pain is not a healthy indicator for timing dental care. At that point, it's often way too late.

( ) Myth 16: "Losing one tooth and not replacing it is not a big deal."

Wrong again. If you lose even one tooth, you can greatly reduce your chewing ability. The teeth around that gap drift that way, leaving their natural "utility zone," and are re-purposed for a job they are not perfect for.

( ) Myth 17: "Dentures work just as well as natural teeth."

No, they don't. With your natural teeth, you can put enough pressure to chew through some pretty tough stuff. In fact, common bite or chewing forces range from 25 to 75 lbs per square inch. And back teeth, when needed, can apply up to 250 lbs per square inch.

And dentures? Dentures generally function at about 25% of normal chewing function. That's right, 75% less. Unless a person's teeth are painful, rotting, or moving, healthy teeth versus dentures are two different worlds.

Over a fifteen year period of wearing dentures, chewing ability deteriorates to 5 lbs of biting pressure. Talk about changing what you can chew! Some people become true dental cripples.

( ) Myth 18: "I don't need regular dental visits."

Your teeth are not self-healing. We wish they were. Dentists and dentistry have long fought for preventive health care. We are justifiably proud of our efforts in the war to battle decay and to teach the public the value of oral health.

The reality is that when teeth are ignored, they'll get worse until they can no longer be ignored.

I still get patients who consistently put off their oral health, time after time. Often these patients come back to us later on after they've had all their teeth removed and had dentures, saying "Please, can you fix me." The reality is that most of the time we can, but at an exponentially higher fee than would have been required if we had been able to fix their real teeth.

"I'll just wait until it hurts, breaks, falls out, or gives me trouble." As a solution, it isn't a solution. I'm still amazed at what people will do for their oral health versus their car or their house or a piece of clothing.

So, "I'll just wait," is like saying "I'm just going to let the bomb blow up before I stop the problem." You wouldn't dare let a bomb go off in a house if you can take the bomb away and have the house still stand. That's what people do when they say, "I'll just wait 'til later." Boom.

And, as many people find out the hard way - it is nearly inevitable that when someone keeps putting off dealing with a dental problem, that problem will flare up at the worst possible time in their life: on a trip, at a business meeting, at an important social gathering, at a funeral, at a wedding or a birthday party.

Ever wonder why that happens? Your body's ability to deal with the chronic stress of the dental problem decreases when afflicted with the added stress of the event.

The delay will make you pay. Who needs the added stress of severe dental problems at the worst possible time? No one.

❨❩ Myth 19: "I can save money if I just put off the dental work."

Putting off dental care can be deadly. Because you suffer no pain at first, some people think they are "getting away with it" or they are "smart enough to know when I really need it." Bad Ideas.

If you are putting off needed care, say hello to trouble. It is coming. Tooth loss and vastly increased expenses are the natural consequences of the delay.

This problem starts with the idea that dental care is elective! No it is not. Dental care should be a regular part of your health care.

Often these delays come from people voting with their pocketbooks. I realize that most people don't budget money for their dental health. It's a shame. It just isn't up there with all the other insistent demands of life and living. Perhaps that will change as people start to realize the connection between their oral health and their overall health.

❨❩ Myth 20: "I've been told I couldn't have implants."

Implants have become the new standard of care for replacing missing teeth. Why? Because they work. Implants don't get decay, and they help to conserve tooth structure on natural teeth that can be left untreated. Moreover, dental implants preserve bone in the jaws and face.

Bone loss causes people to age prematurely, get wrinkles before they are due, and leads to dental handicaps you don't want to endure. The majority of the time, a patient can and should have implants as the preferred method of replacing missing teeth. Any dentist worth his salt will tell you the same.

Most of the time when I hear a patient say, "My other dentist told me I couldn't have implants," it means their dentist didn't know how to perform implant procedures. Dental implants are generally the best long-term solution for replacing missing teeth.

( ) Myth 21: "I don't have to fill out my health history completely at the dentist because my health history doesn't really matter; this is just a dentist."

Your health history does have an effect on the medications we use, how you are treated, and what therapies are prescribed for you.

So, your health present and past does matter. You are wise to answer every question on your health history fully.

If you take a number of medications, one of the best things you can do is make a list of your medications and bring your list in with you at every visit.

( ) Myth 22: "My dental insurance will pay for it all."

Unlike medical insurance, dental insurance has an annual limit. It is a partial benefit plan. It's designed to give you some coverage for what we call "maintenance dentistry." It was never designed to be a pay-all, but people confuse it with medical insurance. It is not the same.

Dental insurance does help, but it was only designed for the simplest type of dentistry that there is. The big problem is the annual limit, which is typically around the $1,000 to $2,000 range these days. That annual limit hasn't kept up with inflation. If it had, it would be closer to $5,000 or $6,000 a year or more.

Fully one third of the people who have dental insurance don't use it, which is sad. Dental insurance can be a great aid to a lot of people, and it's our job to help you get every last nickel coming to you from your dental insurance. Just don't count on dental insurance to pay for everything. It doesn't work that way.

◖◗ Myth 23: "If my insurance doesn't cover it, it must not be needed."

No, this isn't how it works. Dental insurance benefits are purchased by an employer from a dental insurance provider. And just because a particular service isn't covered doesn't mean it's not therapeutically needed; it just means that the employer did not purchase it from the dental insurance benefit company, or that the dental insurance benefit company doesn't offer it.

Often I hear a patient tell me, "My insurance said that your fee isn't usual, customary and reasonable" - not a good thing to hear from your insurance agency, as it often drives a wedge between you and your dentist, and it shouldn't be this way at all.

Of course, the dental insurance company point of view is, "We want X number of dollars from the employer for every employee that's covered, and we want to pay the dental provider "X minus" so that we're profitable." Somewhere around 35% of every dental insurance dollar paid goes to the dental insurance provider.

Now, I have nothing against a dental insurance company making a profit; this is entirely normal. But I do have something against this quote, this statement that's made far too often, "Your fees aren't usual, customary and reasonable." How insurance companies derive their fees are varied. You'll have one company that says the fee is X, another one says it's Y, another one says it's Z.

The reality is that on survey of the Academy of General Dentistry, a group of 25,000 plus dentists, 80% of those answering said that insurance companies said their fees weren't usual, customary and reasonable! How is that possible?

Here's something to keep in mind: The quality of care does make a difference. A dentist is a dentist is a dentist is not true.

Don't be surprised if what your dentist wants to do for you doesn't match the benefits the dental insurance company wants to pay. In fact, expect it.

For a dental insurance company, a dentist is a dentist is a dentist. While we all know it's not true, that's how they like to do it. They make everybody into a commodity. In reality, dentistry is a very highly refined personal service that makes a big difference in your life, and, of course, a profitable insurance company wants to lump everybody together. Such is life.

( ) Myth 24: "Dentistry is expensive."

"Yes, it is," and, "No, it isn't."

If you look at the total fees for care, dentistry or what we call "maintenance" or "check-up" dentistry is pretty reasonable. A person over their lifetime can average somewhere between $1,000 and $2,000 per year in caring for their teeth. Yet when a person neglects their teeth, gets partial treatment, or doesn't see a dentist on a regular basis, dentistry does get expensive. It could have been prevented.

So yes, dentistry can be expensive at times, but here's something else to think about: what's the expense of not seeing the dentist? Isn't that much worse!

( ) Myth 25: "If I have bad breath, I'll just use chewing gum. That'll cure it."

No, this is not true. If you have chronic bad breath, there are usually two reasons why. First, you may have a systemic problem with your whole body. Generally, this can be associated with stomach problems or gastric reflux. The other reason for your bad breath that just won't go away is likely gum disease.

There are some people who chew mints to solve the problem. Not a good idea. Chewing mints or gum to conquer bad breath, when done chronically, encourages dental decay. Oh, boy. Try to solve one problem and you get another! The real solution is to treat the gum disease in the first place, and to get a medical check-up to make sure you don't have something wrong with the rest of your body.

( ) Myth 26: "I'll insult the dentist before we start – that will make my visit better"

Here is how it starts:

"No offense, Doc, but I hate the dentist."

Imagine if you were a dentist and heard this comment!

I try to think mercifully when I hear this comment and understand the point of view of the person saying it.

Generally, jokingly, I will make sure I know what their profession is and then I will say, "Well, you know, I've always hated bar owners," or "I've always hated plumbers," or "I've always hated administrative assistants," or something else just to get the joke across. Usually people get the point right away.

When people say, "No offense, Doc, I hate the dentist," they're really saying, "Hey, I've had a bad experience in the past, I don't like being here because of it."

We understand that, and we work to make sure that that experience doesn't replicate itself for you.

Dentistry no longer has to mean difficulty and challenge. It no longer has to be a dread. No, dentistry doesn't have to be that way at all.

If you still feel like you hate the dentist, you've been seeing the wrong dentist. The new technology and techniques that we have available will make you see dentistry in a whole new way.

John's Story

John was a financial consultant. He announced his position when we first met. I never knew what "financial consultant" meant. He told me he helped people plan for their financial futures, make investments and manage risks. He was quite expressive. At age 47, he was well into his career.

"I'm looking for a boost. I've noticed how my best clients look and act. Since I sell insurance and financial services to them, I need to look like them. If I have country bumpkin teeth, then I'll be seen as less competent. And they demand competence.

"Look, I know I'm very good at what I do and I know you are, too. A friend of a friend sent me here. I want my clients to feel good about dealing with me. I've studied all the books on sales and I have taken dozens of courses over the years. I know that how I look and what my smile says about me matters. Donald Trump may have kept his hair the same way, but he got his teeth fixed and now has a beautiful smile. I want one for me," he finished.

He was right, of course. People first evaluate us by how we look. Sure, clothes and hair matter, but your smile dominates their first impression. Studies show that other people make first impressions of us in as little as nine seconds. These first impressions are important because it is human nature to make evaluations about people we meet quickly. When you flash a good looking smile, your first impression rating goes up, way up.

John didn't need nearly as much as the other patients told in stories here. He had taken pretty good care of his teeth. Still, many things were wearing out. His teeth had darkened. We whitened his teeth, did a few crowns in the back to strengthen broken down teeth, and placed conservative porcelain veneers in his smile zone. We removed the blackened, silver, mercury fillings that made him look a bit dark. We also realigned his bite that had gotten off over the years, much like tires get out of alignment, and then wear excessively.

All of that happened three years ago. Today John is an uber-successful financial consultant. He told me at one of his checkups, "Not only does my smile look great, but I feel so much better, so much more confident. It has helped my career. I've had my best three years ever in a row since you fixed me up."

John had also lost weight because he could chew the right foods again. And since his family had a history of type 2 diabetes, his weight loss and better oral health may very well have headed off diabetes.

"When you told me about the relationship between oral health and diabetes, it was news to me. Now I'm grateful that we headed that off at the pass."

Whenever I see John now, whether in the office or out and about at various charity functions, he's always smiling.

"I love my smile. Thank you."

Thank you, John, for allowing us to give you our best care.

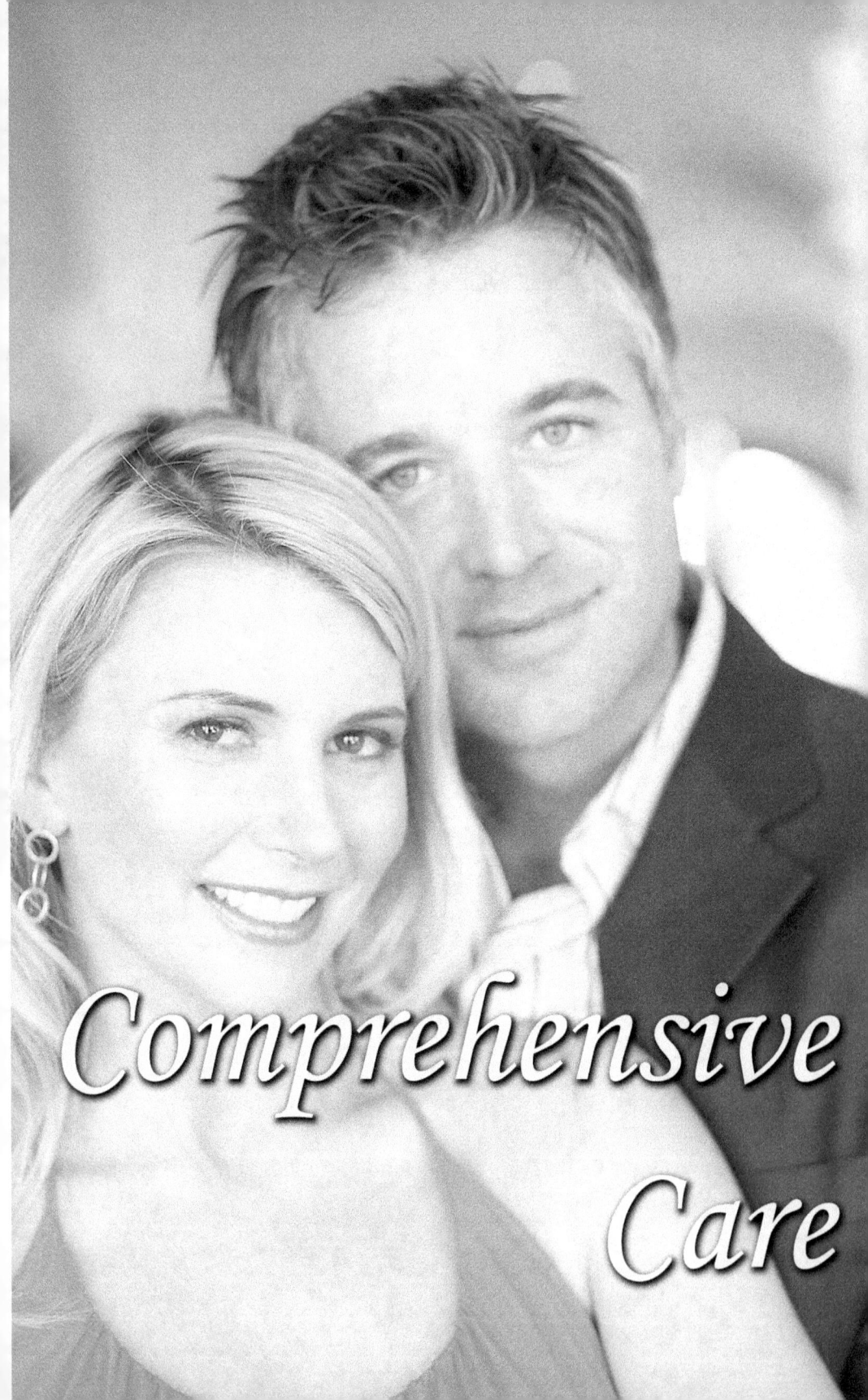

Comprehensive Care

CHAPTER 4

What is Comprehensive Care?

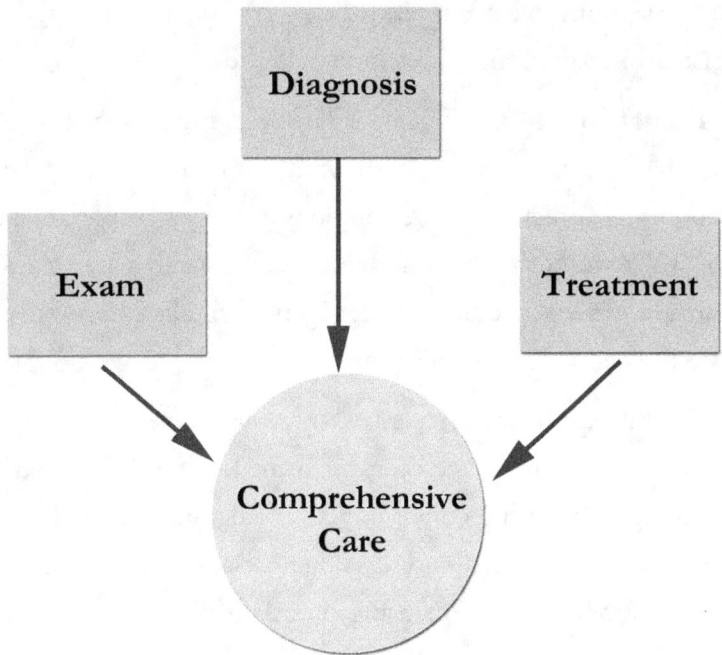

omprehensive care is really all about the type of care that you'd like to have anyway. It is the approach of examining, diagnosing and treating your mouth as a whole, not just as a single tooth or a single problem. It is your best assurance of getting the complete care that ensures you keep your teeth for a lifetime.

Your Chronological Age and Your Dental Age

You can divide a person's dental age into three categories which may be similar to the person's chronological age or may be entirely different. In chronological age, we grow from being a child, to a teenager, to a young adult to an adult to an older adult to a senior to an elder.

The dental ages are youth, adult and elder.

I owe the following word illustrations to Dr. L.D. Pankey, founder of the L. D. Pankey Institute for Dental Education, a post-graduate facility for practicing clinicians in advanced care techniques. He used these descriptions to explain needed care to patients so that they could understand it. I use it here to help you do the same.

Dental "youth" is characterized by no or minimal care other than regular maintenance care. A person with this dental age may have had orthodontic treatment, a few restorations (what lay people call fillings), dental sealants, tooth whitening and wisdom teeth removal. You see this mostly in young adults and teenagers who take care of their teeth and see the dentist on a regular basis.

Dental "adult" is characterized by more problems and treatment. More restorations may have been performed. A tooth may have been lost and replaced with a dental implant or dental bridge. This dental age may have had some gum disease therapy, a root canal or two, some crowns. Cosmetic treatment using porcelain veneers or crowns may have been done.

Incomplete care, partial care or piece-meal patchwork can lead to the next category:

Dental "elder" is characterized by the loss of all teeth and being forced to chew on the gums using removable dentures. THIS IS NOT WHERE YOU WANT TO BE. The older one becomes chronologically, the more difficult this dental age can be. Often having a dry mouth from medications can make wearing removable dentures very uncomfortable and painful.

- The more teeth you have and the better their condition or repaired condition, the 'younger" you are dentally.

- Comprehensive care looks at all of your mouth and teeth and correlates it to all of you as a person.

Chronological Age

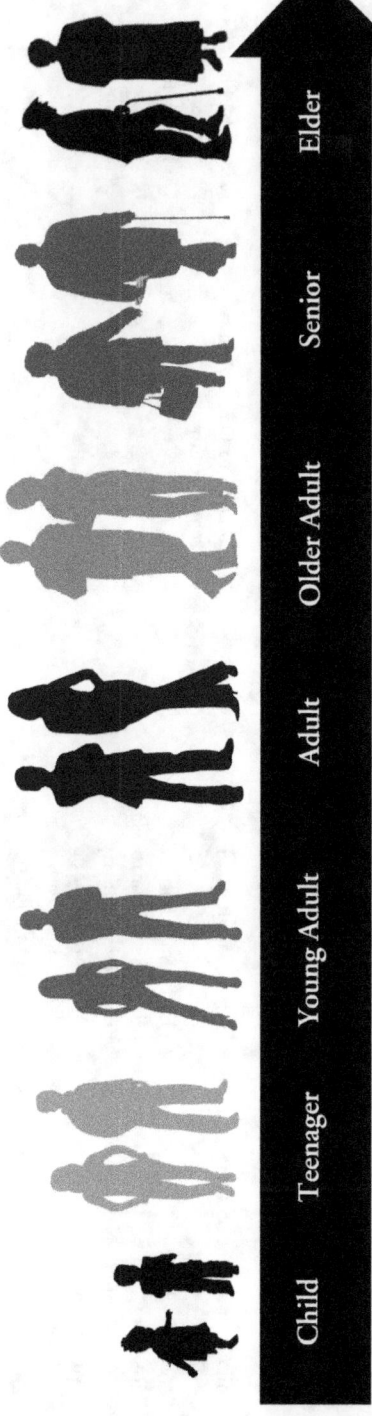

Child | Teenager | Young Adult | Adult | Older Adult | Senior | Elder

Dental Age

Having Teeth ——————————————————————→ Loss of All Teeth

YOUTH

Full Complement of Teeth

Services Include:
Regular Cleanings
Orthodontics
Minor Repairs
Whitening (teenagers)
Wisdom Teeth Removed

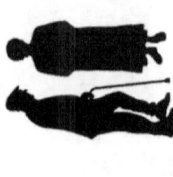

ADULT

Lost a Tooth or a Few Teeth

Early Gum Disease
Repairs - Minor to Major
Cosmetic Dentistry
Adult Orthodontics
Whitening Teeth
Periodontal Plastic Surgery

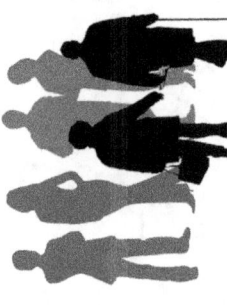
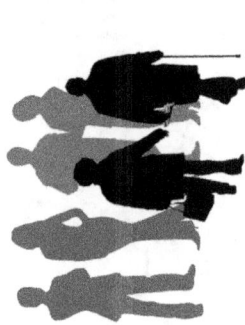

TRANSFORMATION

Restoration to Dental Adult
or Dental Youth

ELDER

Chews on Their Gums

Uses Complete Dentures
(OR Has No Teeth At All -
Dental Cripple)

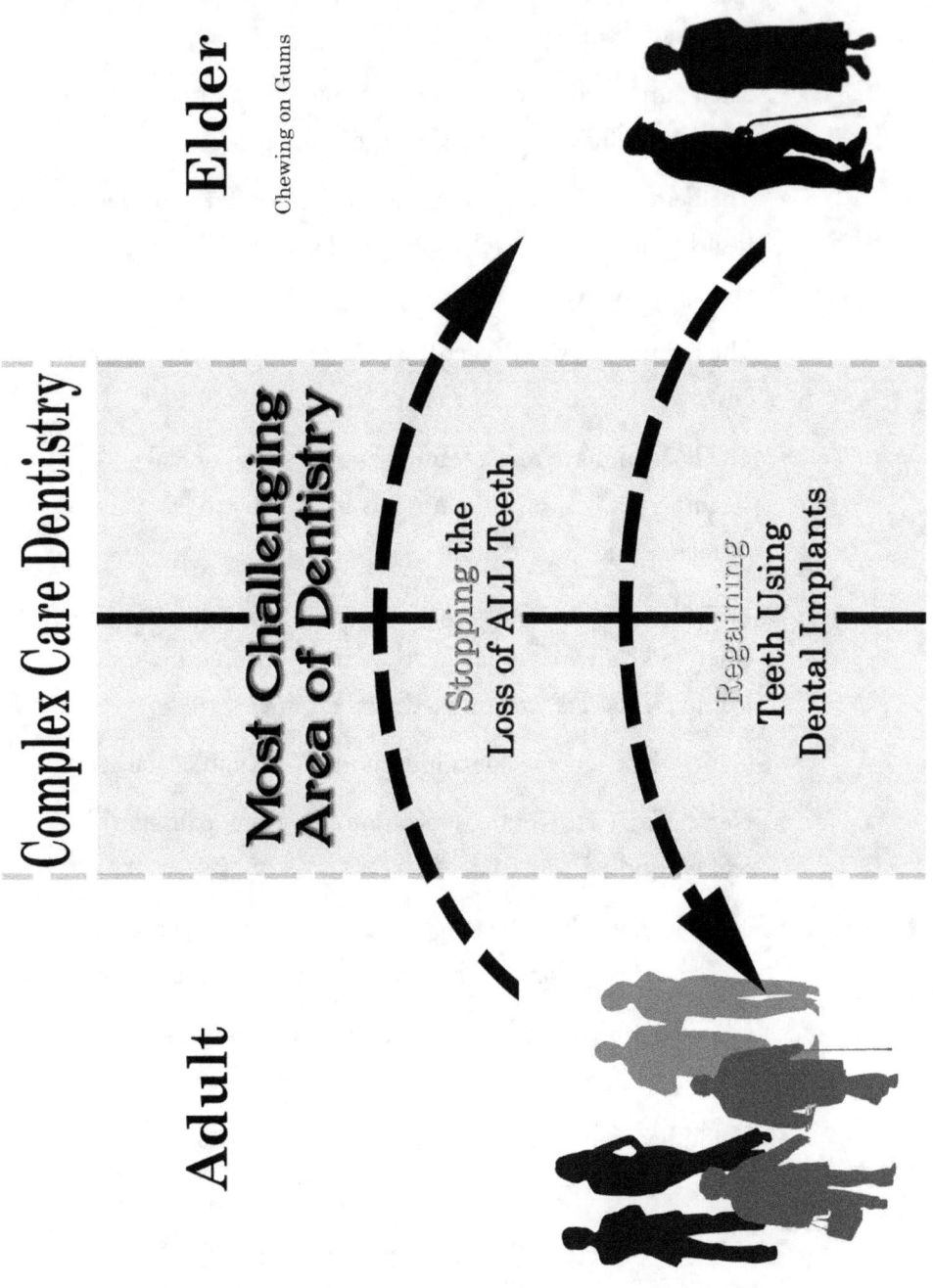

Complex Care Dentistry

Elder

Chewing on Gums

Most Challenging
Area of Dentistry

Stopping the
Loss of ALL Teeth

Regaining
Teeth Using
Dental Implants

Adult

- Your goal should be to stay as young dentally as possible – dental adult or dental youth.

- The younger you are dentally, the younger your entire body seems and this appears to slow the aging process.

- The better the maintenance and prevention for your dental health, the less it "costs" you in the long run and the more youthful you remain.

- The longer you wait to get the care you need, the more it costs you later on and the faster you age dentally.

- The less you have regular, timely professional dental cleanings and exams, the more likely you are to have dental problems and "age" dentally.

- Loss of all teeth as a young adult accelerates aging to dental elder and causes significant, sometimes debilitating bone loss in later years, creating a dental cripple.

- Gum disease is the major culprit in tooth loss and dental aging.

- Neglecting your teeth costs you money, time, pain, health and worsening dental "age."

- The longer you live, the longer you need to keep your teeth. People are living longer. Therefore, you need your teeth longer.

- Chewing on your gums with or without removable dentures can accelerate the aging process.

- If you become a dental elder, act as quickly as possible to get back some teeth that are not removable.

- If you must stay in removable dentures, get the best ones possible. Having really well made dentures improves your appearance, preserves bone longer, and gives you the best fit possible. If you were going to wear only one set of clothes, you'd be pretty darn sure to get the best possible fit, longevity and classic style, right? What do you think you should do with your teeth?

- Dental implants give those who have lost one, a few or all of their teeth a second chance to recover and regain a dental age back to adult.

- The most difficult, challenging areas of dentistry are:

  1. Those charged with stopping the loss of all teeth and thus becoming a dental elder (chewing on the gums.)

  2. Converting a dental elder stage back to a dental adult stage using dental implants.

  3. Challenging cosmetic situations to rebuild smiles as in a complete smile makeover.

  4. Difficult bite situations.

  5. Significant trauma that causes loss of a few or all teeth.

Unlike chronological age, though, dental adult or dental elder can come to you as a chronological youth if there have been enough dental problems.

I have 40, 50, 60 year olds that would still be called dental youths. I also have 20-somethings that are elders, where they've lost all of their teeth, which is sad.

As an adult, as your dental problems worsen and you lose more teeth, you move closer and closer to being an elder. It's in this zone, in the late stage of adult dental treatment that we have the most complex care needs. Failing to treat serious problems differently from everyday dentistry leads to additional tooth loss. The problems of decay, gum disease and your bite mechanism magnify as you lose more and more teeth. One needs an intervention to stop from losing all the teeth. This is complex care dentistry.

The goal of complex care dentistry is to return the person back to a level of health that ensures he won't have to chew on his gums with removable dentures. And this complex care is a whole new way of doing things because now it's far more complicated, far more serious, frankly, more expensive. It's certainly now become an investment in your dental health and is far removed from the "check-up dentistry" being performed for youths and for adults.

Complex care dentistry also includes using dental implants to regain lost teeth and function. This is not for the average dentist without training and experience.

The good news: now, like never before, you have choices. You can stop the progression of losing all your teeth by using dental implants. If you already have removable dentures, you can get dental implants to return you to the state of having teeth again and back into the dental adult stage. When these are done well, you can have the smile of the dental youth.

Make no mistake about it. This is the most challenging and difficult part of dentistry requiring a high degree of skill, training and experience. It is wholly different than check up dentistry found in dental youth and early dental adult stages.

Check-up dentistry costs less, takes less time, is easier to get done, is comprised of fewer visits, etc.

Complex dentistry is more difficult, the fees are exponentially higher, and requires more visits. Complex dentistry requires all the science and arts that we have as dentists combined together to provide you with the care you need to help you keep your teeth for a lifetime.

In other words, complex dentistry is required when your teeth get so bad you need a whole different level of care.

Comprehensive care is the type of care that helps you maintain your optimal dental condition, no matter what stage of dental life you are in. If you're a youth or if you're the parent of a youth, then it is doing all the things that should be done to help that young person keep their teeth for a lifetime.

Comprehensive care also applies to adult care, from replacing a missing tooth if it's lost, to working with a bite problem. And it deals with and eliminates problems that increase the potential for losing teeth.

Comprehensive care also includes complex care dentistry where we take the best of what we have to offer, whether it's gum therapy, bite therapy, cosmetics, implant therapy, and smile design, and use them together to save or recreate healthy teeth.

There are really four reasons why people get in trouble with their teeth.

Reason #1

Dental decay, the old culprit that we have long known to be a problem. Thank goodness, dental decay in general is on the decline. Even today we are making new discoveries about decay. There are at least 32 acid creating, decay causing bacteria and there are five more probable ones. That's a little scary, isn't it?

Reason #2

The second is gum disease, also known as periodontal disease. With what we know about gum disease today and its effect on the rest of the body, gum disease is something we can no longer ignore. It has the potential to lead to your demise.

Reason #3

Stress. The stress caused by the way your teeth come together (occlusion) or body problems has an effect on your teeth. Your dental bite is also known as your dental occlusion – how your teeth meet and function. Your occlusion is influenced by teeth positions, jaw joints (known as temperomandibular joints), muscles of the face, head and neck, muscle activity, oral habits, your chewing mechanism and how much force you put on your teeth either from bite forces or clenching and grinding.

A mismatched bite can be deadly to the longevity of your natural teeth and any dental work. Few people know if they are clenching or grinding since it often happens while sleeping. Usually your dentist can help you discover this. This bite problem may give you no pain at all, yet accelerate wear on your teeth by 10-20 times! The big majority of people who clench or grind have no idea they do it!

When your bite is "off" it requires you to accommodate to the mismatched position. We have seen long term headaches disappear when the bite forces were equalized and normalized for a person.

Reason #4

Systemic problems can affect your dental health also. GERD, also known as GastroEsophogeal Reflux Disease can breakdown the teeth rapidly, increase decay and cause a tooth loss epidemic. All manners of systemic conditions and medications can dry the mouth, alter the immune capacities of the mouth and worsen gum disease and the ability to heal. Diabetes is among the worst culprits, increasing gum disease problems and increasing tooth decay.

Comprehensive care is about dentistry that is predictable. Dentistry that's long-lasting. It takes into account everything in your mouth and your life as factors in designing the right kind of dental care for you. It considers your medical and dental history, as well as your present health, needs, wants and concerns.

We know, for example, if we're going to treat you comprehensively that we need to understand what your past dental experiences have been, be they good, bad or indifferent.

And something for you to realize, if you've had a bad dental experience in the past... it doesn't have to be that way anymore. In fact, old-fashioned dentistry is really a thing of the past. Today, you can get things done more quickly, more comfortably, with better results and greater longevity than ever before with little to no discomfort.

Comprehensive care always starts with an interview of what your expectations are, a review of your history dentally, medically and emotionally. It's taking a look at the whole of you, not just the mouth of you in determining what is the right care specifically for you and all your uniqueness.

Oftentimes when there is significant work to do, we go beyond a regular dental checkup into what we call a complete dental physical. A complete dental physical is a thorough work up consisting of a series of photographs, multiple x-rays, molds of your teeth, facial evaluation, gum disease check and myriad other things that we do diagnostically to gather information. We do this so that we can make sure that all treatment that should occur, does occur.

The more problems you have, the more you need a complete dental physical. Just like when you go to the medical doctor – you can get a check-up for a specific problem, or you can get a complete physical. That complete physical will include a whole host of x-rays, blood tests, and heart checks like a cardiogram. We do something similar with the complete dental physical, but with different tests.

The goal is to leave no stone unturned so we can know your case by heart and know what your particular dental reality is. The goal is optimal treatment designed just for you.

Part of becoming a smart dental consumer is knowing your present level of dental health. Our process in performing a complete dental exam and physical is so you can gain that understanding. That way we can match your care to your needs in an optimal way.

In my office, we try to think in terms of what we call "thirty year treatment plans." Which means whatever we do, we try to give it the capacity or possibility of lasting thirty years. We can't guarantee that it will last that long, but we feel it is our duty to give our patients dental care that has the possibility of lasting that long with proper care and maintenance.

Unfortunately, I see a good deal of dental work done that almost seems as if it's designed to fail within a few years.

When we're doing dentistry, we're not dealing with disposable razor blades. What do I mean by that? Well, Gillette and Schick and all those other manufacturers of razor blades figured out long ago that they could give you the razor blade handle for free because they were going to charge you for the disposable razor blades. Once you have the handle, you'll be paying for blades for a very long time. Dentistry done well should not be like that. We design our care so it can last.

We like to use a concept that has helped structures through-out history last for a long time. The roads, buildings and aqueducts made hundreds of years ago that are still standing were built with the **concept of over-engineering**. These ancient engineers knew that they had to build structures that could withstand weather, man and father time. They had to build structures that were over-engineered so that the stresses of use would not weaken the materials and cause the structure to fall. It was too costly to have it fail before its time.

Today, most modern bridges and buildings meant to last are built with these concepts in mind. Take, for example, a modern bridge over an interstate highway. Smart engineers build it so it can withstand five times normal weights and stresses it most likely will face from the pounding of trucks and cars crossing it. This is the insurance that it will last.

All materials wear out over time. The combined weights of the vehicles, forces of wind and rain, normal wear and tear, even gravity weaken structures over time. When a structure is built to withstand five or ten times the normal load bearing capacity, the stresses of use are minimal. The bridge lasts for tens or even hundreds of years.

We do the same as oral engineers and doctors. We over-engineer your dentistry so that it can last many years, even decades. We create the capacity for it to withstand the biomechanical stresses of everyday chewing and smiling and living. This is why we think in terms of thirty years of service or more.

The problem of engineering for "just the right amount" is what happens when the work is stressed beyond normal. Will it fail? Are you willing to risk it? Would you buy an insurance policy that was good only half the time? What if you got unlucky and the day you needed it, you weren't insured?

We don't want to count on luck. We want to be sure. Don't you?

Over-engineering does take more time, effort and energy and does cost a bit more, and the result is long lasting dental work that looks good, feels good, lasts and gives you piece of mind. The value of that is immense to you, wouldn't you agree?

Unfortunately, we see much dentistry outside our offices done for expedient reasons that will be lucky to last for five years. It is typically under-engineered. The sad truth is that unless you are a smart dental consumer who knows what to ask you could be fooled into thinking you were getting something you were not.

Incidentally, a lot of dental insurance companies will repay for things every five years. On the one hand, that is very good, and very bad on the other. It doesn't take a math genius to figure out that you're better off paying for something once and having it last a very long time than having it replaced every five years. Unfortunately, the latter occurs far too frequently.

So, don't fall into the trap of "Scotch Tape dentistry." It binds parts together and maybe doesn't look too bad, but it's a classic example of under-engineering care that's destined to fail, often at the worst possible time.

Now, you should expect something else from comprehensive care. It will cost you more than five-year or "Scotch Tape" care. That should make sense. Remember that thirty-year care: 1) in the long-run, is cheaper, 2) feels better, 3) looks better, 4) works better over time, 5) lasts longer and 6) gives you peace of mind. Isn't that what you want?

It is common for an individual to under-estimate the fees associated with comprehensive care when there are major problems, often by a third to a half of what it will actually be. A common mistake is to compare check up dentistry to complex care dentistry. They aren't the same. And you don't want check up type dentistry done when you have complex care needs, that could lead to very unsatisfactory results.

Understand this too: your dentist should understand the difference between check-up care and complex care. Comprehensive care involves doing the right thing no matter what your dental age is. It includes both check up care dentistry and complex care dentistry. Complex care deals with very difficult situations cosmetically, functionally and otherwise.

Comprehensive care is at once a better solution, and the right solution, and if you would ask any dentist what type of dentistry they would personally prefer, you'd almost always hear, "I'd like to have comprehensive care."

Hopefully, you don't find many dentists who need complex dentistry, but if they do, you can bet they want the best dentistry possible because they know the difference.

Summary

Comprehensive care dentistry is a way of diagnosing and treating dental cases so that optimal care is performed whether it is check up type dentistry or complex care dentistry. It is a way of looking at you and your oral condition as a whole, not as one tooth at a time.

If you have complex care needs, be sure that you get someone trained in complex care and its many thousands of nuanced methods so you can be assured that the right kind treatment fits your condition. Over- engineering is one of the best ways possible for you to ensure that your work has the biomechanical capacity to last for years and years.

As you might guess, there is far more to dental care than just these parts. There are also biologic concerns of the tissues, cosmetic and smile design components and bifunctional parameters of the chewing mechanism. Your dental success also requires for you to be a partner in your care. This includes your home care and your regular professional hygiene maintenance visits in your office. Don't worry. We can make it all understandable and easy for you.

Frank's Story

For Frank, his teeth had never been a priority. He had always been so busy. He had dutifully paid for all three kids to get braces and his wife went to the dentist regularly. Now the kids were out of the house, he decided to take a more careful look at his appearance. It was one of those regular mornings before work when, after brushing his teeth, he stood there and looked at them.

Frank told us, "I'm not sure why I really noticed them that morning, but I did. And I did not like what I saw. My smile was, shall we say tattered. My teeth had darkened. They were quite yellow. My old dental work was showing its age. I had thought my teeth were OK. I mean acceptable, at least. They really weren't. That was when I decided to do something.

As a big league executive, Frank was at a place professionally where he needed every edge he could garner. Freshly minted MBA's were joining his company every year. Although these were two and three levels below him, he knew they would be his competition in the future. Already his former colleague, Richard, had reached the C-level position he coveted.

"It dawned on me later that morning after I had really noticed my teeth that Richard had had his teeth fixed. He received the nod of promotion instead of me. I knew that results of performance mattered, but I think his new smile gave him the edge I didn't have. I mean we were both pretty equal otherwise."

Frank got his smile makeover done. Moreover, we found an oral health- total body health connection to Frank's pre-diabetes and snoring. (It is estimated that over 57 million adults over age 40 are pre-diabetic. Pre-diabetes means that one's fasting blood sugar is in the range of 101 to 125. 126 and above is considered diabetic.)

"I wish I had this done years ago. I know it has made a real difference for me. I feel so much better about myself. My wife says I look fifteen years younger. Within a few months, my promotion came through too. Now Richard and I are colleagues once again. And my wife is much happier now that my snoring is no longer a problem. My M.D. says the diabetes screening was a good catch. I've even lost weight."

Frank made a difference for himself that ended up helping him get a promotion (and the increase in pay that comes along with it). His wife told us privately that not only can she get a good night sleep, but also likes having her husband smile all the time. He is happier… and so is his wife.

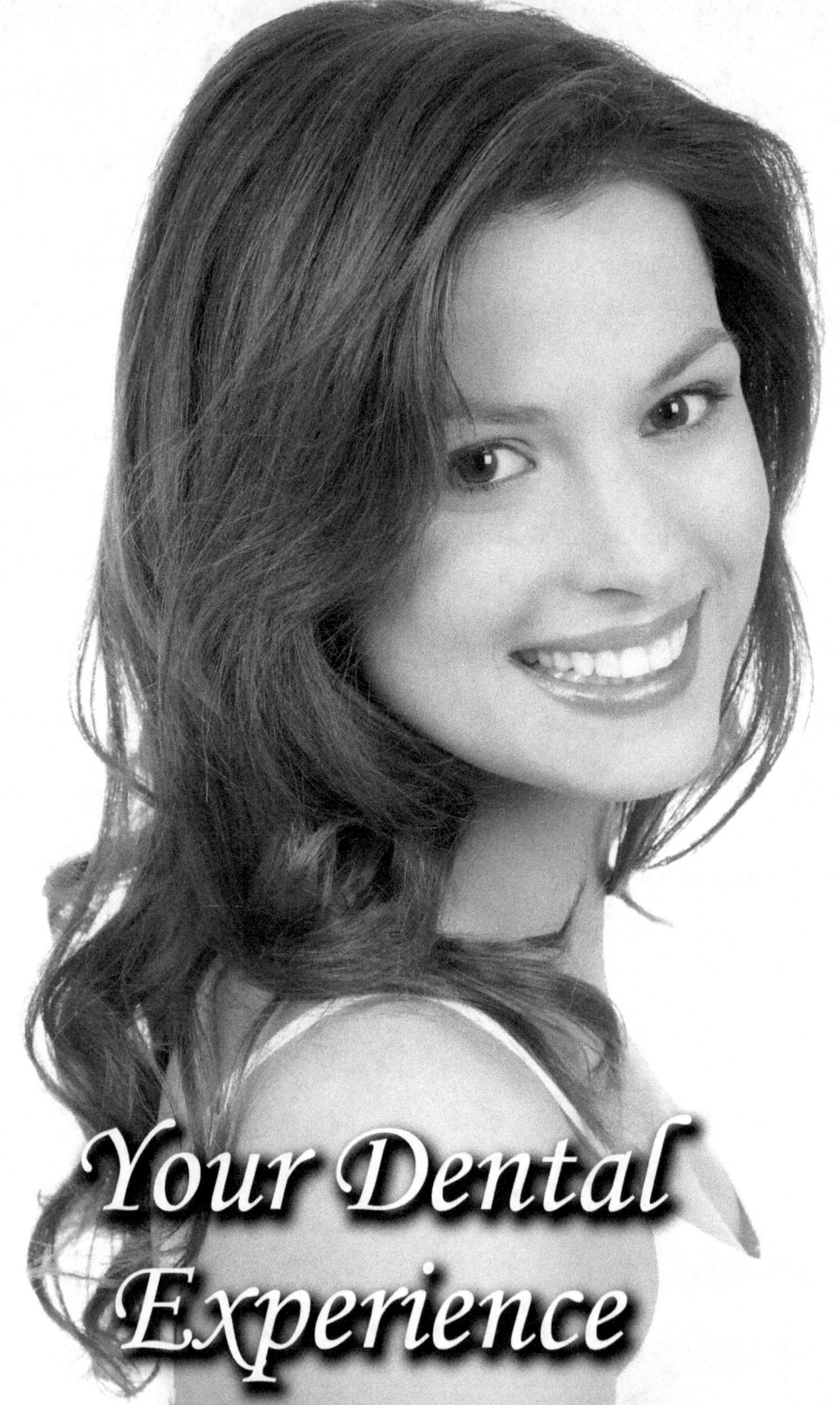

Your Dental Experience

CHAPTER 5
Your Dental Experience

You might be surprised why people don't go to a dentist on a regular basis. Let me give you a hint. It is not because of anxiety or fear or a previous bad experience.

The number one reason? The failure to see a need! I could hardly believe it when I read this survey many years ago. This indicates a failure of my profession and health care in general to make a specific point of what should be regular dental visits to prevent the loss of teeth and keep the public smiling.

After reading about the public perception of the reasons why dentists want patients to return at least twice a year for maintenance and professional cleanings, I was really surprised.

What was the reason that the public believed dentists wanted them to come in regularly?

One particular survey said because dentists wanted to make money. Color me shocked. At first, anyway. Then disappointed.

As a dentist, I know that we make precious little money from the regular maintenance care. The real reasons are because it is our duty to advise on the best possible care and regular maintenance every few months are part of that best possible care. Regular visits for preventive care is one the most cost effective ways to keep your teeth and reduce dental costs.

If one would really consider it, the profession of dentistry has been at the forefront of preventive care since the 1950's. Many of us have worked without pay to ensure that community fluoridation was in the water supply, often against significant odds.

What is the number two reason that people don't come to a dentist? A previous bad dental experience.

Many people see dentistry as a discretionary expense rather than a health care investment. Sadly, most just doesn't know enough to make a good decision.

I'm confident that after reading this book, at least you will be.

Let's begin by discussing reason number two – the bad dental experience. As children, many boomers and older folks had a bad experience at the dentist's office as a child.

Most children don't think particularly clearly and or logically, and don't understand most of what's going on. But they do understand their parents, often one of whom was likely to tell them "not to be afraid" of the dentist.

So, what does a child do when it's told not to be afraid or don't worry? The child becomes afraid and worries.

It's no one's fault. It just is.

At that time, dentistry was not as technologically adept, nor was it as aware of emotional needs as today's modern dentistry. Dentistry was still learning a lot.

Our medical brethren were putting people to sleep for procedures for which we were using local anesthetics - often with agents that didn't numb very well.

No wonder people didn't like it. No wonder people had bad memories. Heck, dentists didn't like it either!

Some still have those memories today.

I've had many a patient enter my practice say, "Look, Doctor, I know I shouldn't be afraid. I know things are different, but I just had a bad experience when I was a little kid."

"Well, how old were you?"

"I think I was 5." This came from an adult age forty-seven!

They're illogical and they still continue to impact the life of those affected.

Let's understand why bad experiences are remembered. When you have stress, you're fearful or you have pain, the body secretes what we doctors call epinephrine, or what the public calls adrenalin.

Adrenalin is the fight or flight hormone that prepares the body to either fight or flee. As a child, there's not much you could have done in the way of fleeing or fighting. And your parents and the dentist were bent on getting you through the procedure.

That experience of anxiety, turning into fear, coupled with pain, mixed with adrenalin burned those memories into the neurons of the mind. Because they were burned in, they are still there. And they can be overcome. We help patients get past those early memories every day.

If you have had those bad memories, know this: It's a new time. Old fashioned dentistry is gone. The dark times of imagined or real dental dungeons, where you never knew what was going on, it always hurt and the whole thing was difficult, are gone.

In dentistry today we work to make your visits as simple, and as comfortable as possible. Our materials and technologies make things far easier. And we have new understandings of how people think and deal with stress. We know how the brain responds to emotional signals, so we can be more comforting. The result is a very different dental experience than times of old.

Here is how you can participate with your dentist to make it a Positive Dental Experience:

- Tell your dentist what you want. Share what kind of things you'd like to see, and how you'd like your dental experience to feel.

- Ask the questions you want to have answered. It is only fair that you get your questions answered, right?

- Ask enough questions so you understand enough to make a decision.

- Don't put off dentistry that you need to have done because it will cost you in the long run.

- Do work with your dentist as a partner. Give your complete health history.

- Tell your dentist how your dental visits have been for you in the past.

- Tell your dentist what you really envision for your smile and your dental health.

- Do understand that your dental decisions have health enhancing or disease enhancing effects on the rest of your body.

- If you're a parent with a child, teeth have an enormous cumulative effect on their lifelong health.

- Tell the dentist if you need to get up and move around.

- Let your dentist know if you feel any discomfort at all.

- Let your dentist know if you need to use the restroom, adjust the chair, or get better support for your neck.

We all really want a Positive Dental Experience. It's interesting, there's no dental insurance code for dental experience, yet a positive one can mean all the difference between a big bright beautiful smile and shunning dentistry forever.

Gratefully, it's a new day. "It ain't like it used to be". Thank God. Welcome to the no lecture zone, no finger wagging, no reprimanding, treat-you-like-a-human-being dental practice. They're really out there, and one of the goals of this book is helping you find them.

Towards that end, one of the things we do at our offices is design and decorate differently. What you see does count, as well as what you hear. So we provide iPods and CD's so you can listen to what you want.

We've created what we call an aesthetic design. What's an aesthetic design mean? It means a design as it is defined by architecture, a place that feels good to be in. That's why we designed our office the way it is, so it can feel right- like the right kind of space.

The Chinese have a name for this. They call it feng shui, a system of design that allows a person to feel comfortable and strong in a space.

We even changed the smells. We removed the materials that don't smell good.

We changed the taste of many of the materials. We're not saying we're a restaurant, but we do work to make the taste you encounter here as pleasant as possible.

Certainly, we work to have a light touch so your experience of working with us is as good as it can be.

Your friendly gentle dentistry is one of our goals, as it is with all the better dental offices out there.

Likewise, better dentists tell patients what they should expect during their visit, because being able to predict what's going to happen, helps reduce anxiety or outright fear, and creates a more comfortable atmosphere for everyone. It gives one a better sense of control.

We've changed our technology. We have all sorts of gadgets and goodies, all sorts of things that help you get more comfortable. We believe dentistry is better for it.

And just as importantly, we dentists have improved the way we communicate. At one point, dentists were so busy just trying to conquer decay that they had no time to work on the finer points of chair-side manner. But decay is not the problem it once was, which has allowed dentistry to become far more patient-focused and treatment to become much easier.

The right dentist for you should want to make your visit a Positive Dental Experience...so you'll want to come back.

In return, today's better dentists will:

- Explain what they do.
- Show you why they need to do it
- Go to great efforts to make sure that you're comfortable by performing the most modern techniques
- Apply the latest technology to give you the longest lasting results possible.

Our job as care providers is to give you predictable, positive experiences. Your job is to help us by partnering in your dental experience so you can be comfortable, so you can be happy with the care that you get, and so you feel a sense of control over what's going on.

We're going to give you that control to the degree that you need it so you can feel comfortable.

Quick story: I once had a prominent businessman fly to see us who was terribly uncomfortable with getting his dental work done. To conquer this, all we had to do was give him some control. He had tried sedation dentistry, but even that didn't alleviate his fear.

Although sedation dentistry is "just the trick" for many people, for this guy it wasn't. He needed to feel he could control the experience so it could fit with what he needed emotionally. We gave him that control, and as a result he finally got the dentistry done that he'd been putting off for 20 years. Today, the guy has a big, bright, beautiful smile and smiles all the time, before he used to hide it.

For many people anxious about seeing the dentist, just telling you that you no longer need to be fearful isn't going to be enough.

The new reality is that you no longer have to be fearful. That day is gone. Good Riddance.

A new day is here. Hurray for us all!

As you read the next chapters we believe you'll discover reasons to see a new kind of dentist; reasons powerful enough to compel you to come in and find out for yourself.

Bill's Story

Bill was a Fortune 500 executive who came to us with a "list of concerns." From the beginning, he seemed to be far more aware than most patients. Somehow his knowledge just didn't match the time pressure that is so often associated with high level executives. When could he have found the time to become so knowledgeable?

He gave me his list when I asked why he was here. The last one was telling.

"Why am I here? Let me tell you why," Bill began with his friendly directness. "Number one, in my position I have to be the representative, the face of my company to the public. I meet with government officials, shareholders, financial analysts, board members, you name it. I have to look the part, the better I look, the easier it is to be persuasive. I have to influence a lot of people to our way of thinking. I'm somewhat of a celebrity and as a celebrity, my appearance means a lot for me and my company."

He was right. Now I was wondering how he came to learn all of this. He continued...

"Number two, I realize that my teeth are vital to my health. I didn't use to think this. Now I know better. My cardiologist has been after me for a while to get my teeth fixed because he told me that the health of my mouth affects the health of my heart."

(This Fortune 500 CEO was smart. Maybe his ability to listen and learn helped bring his success, I thought.)

"Number three, I want to live a good long time. I want to see my grandchildren grow up. I want to help them. I was so busy when my own kids were growing up that I missed out on a lot. I missed their birthdays, school events, games. I missed too much. I really regret it now. So I want to take charge of my own health."

(Although empirically derived, I have found that my patients who do get their teeth fixed and keep their mouths healthy do live longer- and with a better quality of life.)

He went on...

"Number four, I don't have time to waste so I need someone like you that can get things done quickly without sending me all over to see a multitude of other dentists."

Well, he was right again. My curiosity was now just too great. His announcements of why he was here were just too well put together, so direct.

I said, "So how did you find out about all of this? You know, not one in a hundred patients comes in here knowing what you know. I doubt you researched it yourself."

He nodded yes to the last statement.

"So how did you find out about these things," I prodded. He smiled.

"Every good man has a good woman behind him. My wife researched all this on the internet and would read it to me while we were in bed at night before going to sleep."

Hooray for wives who care and husbands who listen, I thought.

It is estimated that wives and mothers of the world help make the vast majority of all healthcare decisions and then direct those that they love where to go and what to do. Dr. Mom lives.

"So how did you find us? You are located several states away and obviously came here at no small expense," I inquired.

"Well Doc, you were referred to me by another one of your patients. My wife asked around and her friend insisted I should come here," he said with a certain expectancy of tonality as if to say 'I hope you are worth it.'

I answered the unspoken question. "We have lots of important people like you in our practice so it is common for people to travel great distances to see us. You can rest assured we stand behind what we do. And we'll get your work done in as few appointments as possible. We'll teach you how to keep your mouth clean and what foods to avoid.

"You are obviously a smart and successful man. You've made another wise decision. Are you ready to get started?" I asked.

He nodded.

We went through the rest of our interview, completed our Complete Dental Physical with dispatch.

He needed a lot. It was one of those cases where he was threatened with losing all his teeth had he not acted when he did.

We completed his work over the next months on specially scheduled trips to optimize as much work being done at once as possible. We had to integrate gum treatment, tooth removal, bone grafting, dental implants, smile design, plastic surgery for his gums and crown work for his entire mouth. Not every patient who comes to us from afar needs this much work, but Bill did. We got it done quickly to match his schedule (including meeting his private plane at the airport).

Today, Bill and his wife have retired to their second house in a warm climate. Bill and his wife see their grandchildren a lot – just like he said he would.

Helping people like Bill and the others in the stories told here gives us the professional satisfaction that means so much. We made a difference and that's why we do what we do.

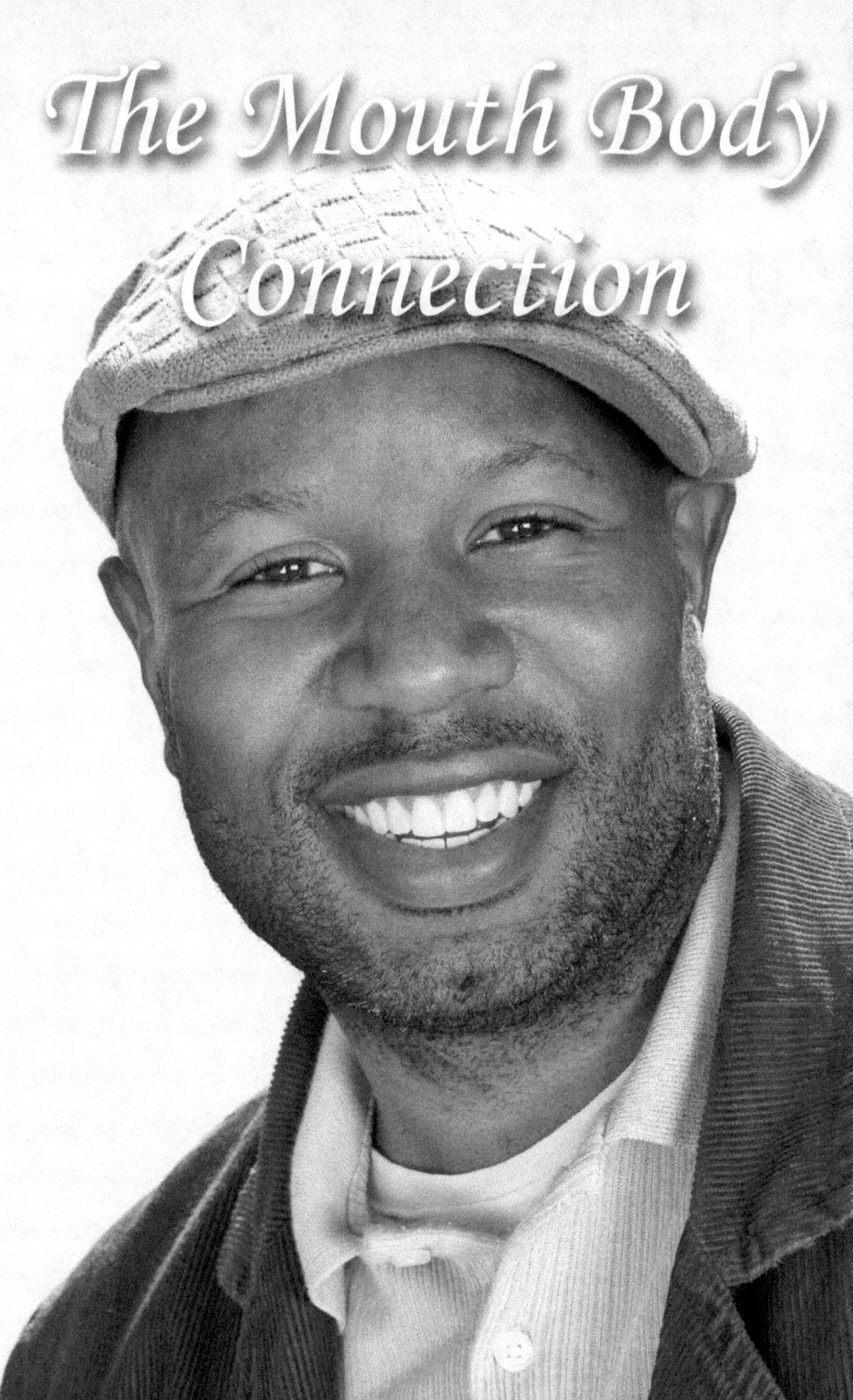

CHAPTER 6
The Mouth Body Connection

T he fact that the health of your mouth affects your body should not come as a shock. The fact that dentists are trained in separate professional schools than physicians and other health care providers means nothing other than dentistry is a specialty of health care.

So, why is there a disconnect?

Why do people have the idea that dentistry doesn't have an effect on their overall health?

Well, I think it's for a number of reasons.

Number one is our medical brethren, particularly physicians, who are not taught that the mouth has much to do with the work they do. In fact, they're taught next to nothing about teeth, gum disease and dental health. They look past the teeth. For many, the body starts at the throat.

The doctors with the fullest understanding are the physicians who are attuned to the interaction between oral health and total body health. Many cardiologists have come to realize that dental disease has a direct effect on the heart and advise their patients accordingly. "Get your teeth fixed and keep them that way," can become life – saving for the heart patient or those who have suffered strokes.

Some endocrinologists now understand that diabetes and dentistry are intimately connected. What makes dental health worse will make diabetes worse, and what makes diabetes worse will make dental health worse. Likewise, improving your dental health makes it easier to control your diabetes.

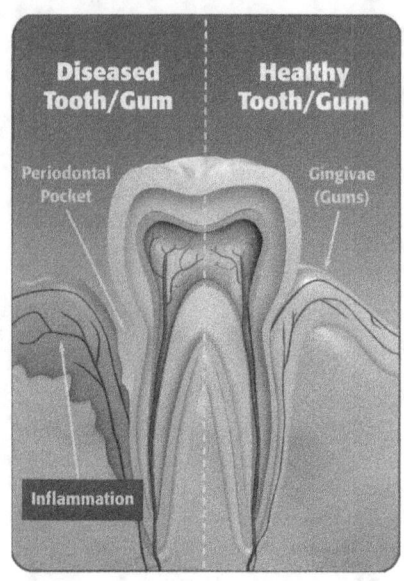

Some orthopedists require their patients to get a clean bill of dental health before they will do significant bone/joint surgery. They learned that lesson the hard way. Poor dental heath with active disease was traced back as a primary reason that some orthopedic surgeries failed.

The second reason for the disconnect is the media. Television, newspapers, magazines, and books largely ignore dentistry as part of the prescription for health. I don't think it's the right idea. I don't know why it's there. I attribute it to physicians' roles of sole arbiters of health in our society.

There's this sort of weird disbelief that people have about the connection between their mouth and their health. But with what we know now, this connection of the oral health with the total body health has never been as clear.

Understand this: infections in your mouth cause inflammation in your body. How so?

If your gums bleed, you have at least a low-grade infection in your mouth. And such an infection in your mouth causes your liver to secrete three things.

Number one, it causes your liver to secrete more cholesterol. The liver is the main source of cholesterol in the body in the first place, and a mouth infection boosts its normal secretion.

Number two, it increases your glucose level, which only makes sense. The body takes inflammation to equal infection. And since the body must fight infection, it produces more glucose for cells to have the strength to make this fight.

Number three, is called C-reactive protein, which we're only beginning to understand. C-reactive protein is an inflammatory marker. Meaning, as inflammation increases, the amount of C-reactive protein increases as well.

A normal measurement for C-reactive protein in health is between 1 and 3. Three is a bit high; less than one is very good. We find that in those with chronic gum disease, the amount of C-reactive protein is directly linked to the severity of the disease.

That is a very bad thing because we know that the higher the C-reactive protein, the more likely you are to have a whole set of problems you want no part of; like heart attack, stroke and diabetes, which is particularly problematic for those with gum disease, because gum disease and diabetes both amplify each other. Diabetes makes the gum disease worse and the gum disease makes the diabetes worse. (Yes, I know I have repeated myself, but it bears repeating.)

The inflammatory response to a gum infection can also affect a pregnant female, increasing the likelihood of premature births and low birth weight babies. Some medical insurance companies have recognized this, too. They provide some dental care for pregnant mothers under the medical insurance because they know it decreases the money they spend to care for these new babies.

Likewise, gum disease increases the risk of developing a number of cancers, including deadly pancreatic cancer; by as much as 59% over someone who does not have significant gum problems.

The bacteria in the mouth can re-seed gastric ulcers by transferring *H. Pylori* from the oral tissue to the gut. This can start the ulcer all over again.

Inflammation in the mouth increases upper respiratory diseases like pneumonia. Breathing those bacteria in from your mouth when you have gum disease is not good for you.

Inflammation in the mouth worsens both osteoarthritis and rheumatoid arthritis. In fact, it has been shown that rheumatoid arthritis sufferers are 400% more likely to have periodontal (gum) disease!

It has an effect on snoring and sleep apnea.

As you are likely aware from your own experience, a large portion of the adult population snores. And approximately 10% of the adult population has some form of sleep apnea. The more severe the sleep apnea, the more it inhibits proper sleep. And we've discovered that lack of sleep alters the secretion of a hormone called leptin, increasing your appetite, creating a direct effect on obesity.

One of the emerging areas of research is inflammation and its effects on your total health. We know that gum disease affects seventy-five percent of the population of North America. This ranges from slight to severe. The more severe the gum disease is, the greater the level of inflammation.

One hypothesis is that diabetes mellitus is a disease **caused** by inflammation. There have been over 1,000 articles written since 2005 on the connection between diabetes and your oral health.

 Go to **www.pubmed.com** and check it out yourself.

Georgia's Story

Georgia came to us at the age of 62. She was just about to retire when she came across some articles on the internet that spurred her visit. Her teeth were in very bad shape.

"Doc, I want to live the rest of my life as long as I can with the highest quality possible.

"I know that keeping my teeth and getting the bad ones out and replacing them with the kind that doesn't come out can make a big difference in both years in my life and life in my years."

Directness again. That is so much better than patients who don't tell us what's really important to them. It is as if hiding health information or their real motivation is a proper test of my care, skill and judgment. It is not. "Telling all" simplifies things for everyone concerned and makes life easier for both the patient and the dentist.

"Georgia, you are right to be concerned," I agreed. "We know that people will need their teeth longer. Over half of those living to age of 60 will live to be in their 90's or longer. And with the strides being made in genetics and genomics, life spans over a hundred are likely. Chances are, you'll need your teeth longer."

Georgia nodded her head in agreement. "I didn't know that, but I do now. I don't plan to retire in the traditional way of my parents. No rocking chair and old folk's activities for me. I plan on being very active in my retirement. I'm going to need my teeth.

"I plan to travel, finally, as much as I always wanted to, and I will volunteer. Who knows, I may even start my own business."

"I want to be able to enjoy my food. You know eating is one of life's special pleasures as you get older, especially when I am eating with the ones I love. Those are special times. I want my quality of my life to be at its highest possible.

"I watched as my parents had to be put in nursing homes. I saw how poorly they were able to eat. Orderlies lost their dentures. I don't want to be like that. I want to be able to live differently from them. I loved them dearly and still miss them. I just don't want to be forced into a situation where I don't get to choose. I know one of the best investments I can make today is to get my teeth in good health and keep them that way. That's why I'm here. I'm ready," She finished.

"Georgia, you are right. You have obviously been looking at this for a long time. I appreciate how you feel."

"Is there anything else I should know?" I was asking because I know that often patients will think of more to say. I want to ensure I cover all of their concerns and answer all of their questions.

"Just this, I know that it will cost a lot. I am in pretty bad shape. I just don't look at it as an expense or unnecessary expenditure. To me, getting my teeth back in good health gives me a second chance. I've denied myself for years for my family. It's time for me."

Georgia was right. And like so many others, she had denied herself for years for the sake of her family.

She continued, "I know that by doing this for me now, I am also doing this for them in the future. I'll be around longer, feeling better, setting an example for them. They don't have my problems. It finally dawned on me that those who don't have problems like mine can't appreciate or even understand why it is so important to me or why it would be this big of an investment."

Georgia had done her homework. Her insights into human nature and the love of her family were obvious. She also realized that no one else could understand her problems like she could. She lived with them every day. She wasn't a complainer and so it was natural for them to question her about doing something now. She didn't tell them all. It was just easier that way, she told me later.

Her family and friends think her new smile has made her look fifteen years younger.

She had lost her husband four years ago. And while not looking for another man, she said she wouldn't mind the companionship of a male friend. After she had her work done, *he found her.* They have been together now for nearly five years. Robert, her new man, told me, "She is just so alive, so upbeat. Her smile says it all. We are really enjoying these years together. She had lost her husband and I had lost my wife. Both died from cancer. Now, together we volunteer for cancer research," he said with pride.

Georgia made a decision for a new smile – it seems it sparked a new life. I can't say that will happen for you, dear reader, but it is a common result.

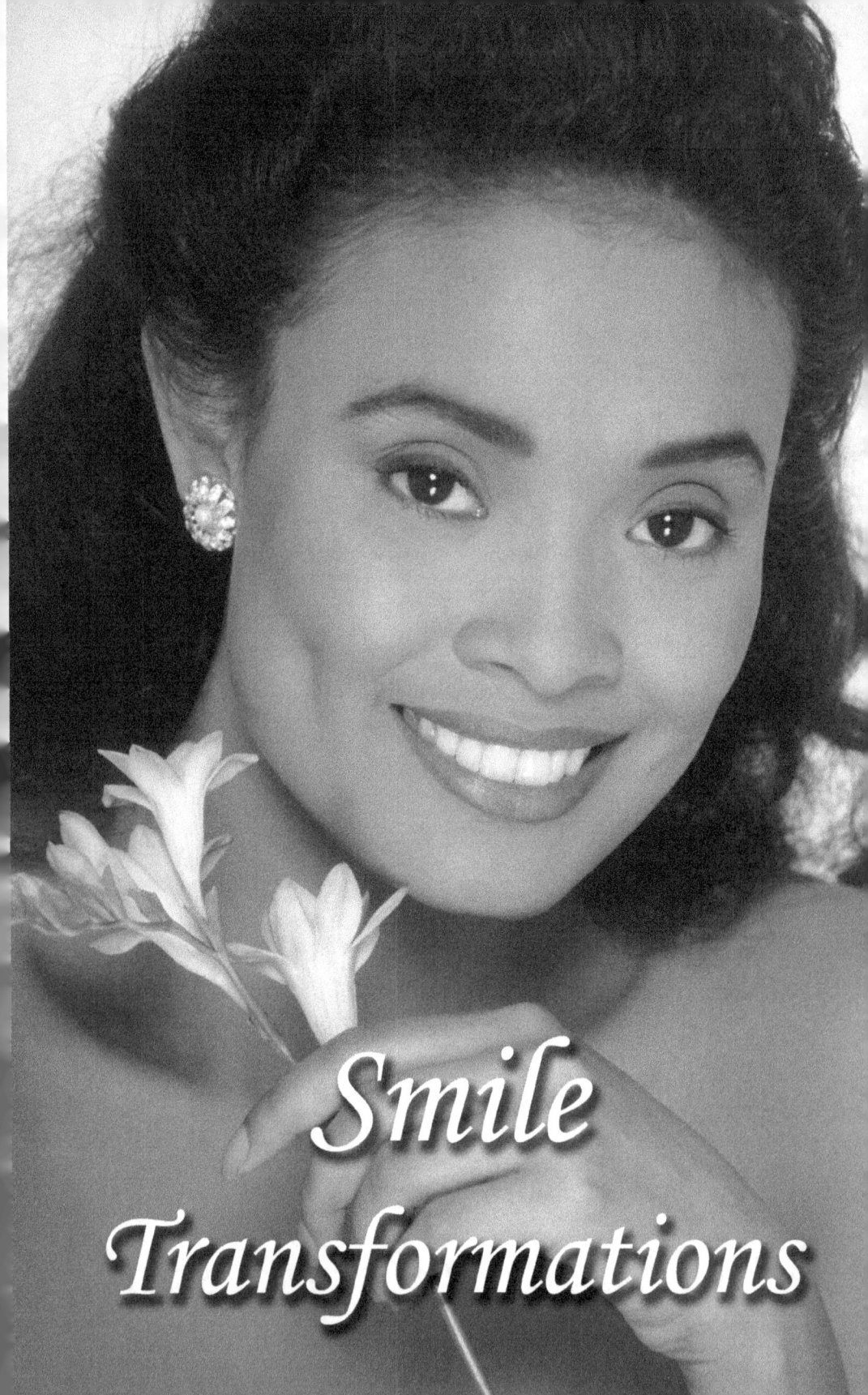

Smile
Transformations

CHAPTER 7
Smile Transformations

As many people travel through life, they get behind, so to speak, on their dental health. For myriad reasons - a failure to see a need, a previous bad experience, financial concerns, paying to get the kids through college and others - they ignore the warning signs. Then one day, they wake up to realize what they have lost.

"Hey, I want my smile back," is the common remark they make when they visit us.

What they are asking for is a smile makeover, what we sometimes call a smile renaissance.

Whether your dental health is a disaster or you just want to look your best, today's dentistry can give you the smile you have always wanted. You can experience your very own version of a smile renaissance. It can have immense effect for you personally.

A smile renaissance can literally transform the way you look. It can make wrinkles, and facial imperfections seem to disappear. If you ever watched the makeover shows on TV, you remember that the dental work often made the biggest difference in how they looked.

A smile makeover or enhancement can create an enormous physical transformation. Who doesn't want a great looking smile?

What you may not take into account is the effect the physical transformation has on the rest of your life. This physical transformation is the first part of what I call the PIES formula. PIES stand for Physical, Intellectual, Emotional, and Spiritual. What happens in one part of your life in any one of those dimensions will usually affect all the other parts.

If you improve your physical appearance, it has a ripple effect. If you look better, you feel better about yourself. Others will likely think you more intelligent, and emotionally, you'll feel better. You may arouse interest of that certain someone you want noticing you. In fact, studies have shown that the better you look, the better others treat you. It's human nature. People inherently know this, that's why they "dress up" for significant events, celebrations and times – so they can look as good as possible.

I've had many of these big problem patients say, "I'm the worst case you've ever seen," and I have to reassure them that they are not. We can help virtually anyone have a good looking smile again and regain their dental health.

Not all dentists are equally qualified to do this kind of work. It takes a lot of training, talent, skill, art and science to do these smile transformations. So make sure that you find someone who is experienced and does this unique type of work on a regular basis. Why? Because it requires us to consider every facet of dentistry, hundreds of considerations, big and small, to properly diagnose and treat cases like these.

We must consider the biology of the teeth and gums, whole body health, the biomechanics of function, the bio-structural integrity of the treatment we are performing, the cosmetic realities and patient concerns to ensure that we build a smile that helps you get your "smile mojo" back. We have to consider your age and stage in life, your chewing habits, diet, jaw joint health and durability requirements of the treatment we will be performing.

We have to ask ourselves, "Given this patient's situation, wants, and needs, what makes the best long term solution?"

Just as importantly, we have to consider how your past experiences have impacted you and what we need to do to help you get past any bad ones.

Often, we will show you your smile changing possibilities before we ever start by showing you how you'll look after the treatment is completed. We do this using a computer program and your photos to simulate just how good your smile can look after we are finished. Most people are surprised at the huge difference. A common comment is, " I had no idea that I could look that good again!" or another one, "I never looked that good even with my old teeth!" While it is but a simulation, usually our patients look better than the simulated smile when we are finished with the actual treatment.

Sadly, some people say, "Well, I'm not sure I'm worth all that. That seems like a lot for me to do."

I understand the feeling. And smile transformations often are a lot of work. But are you worth it? If you believe in yourself and your contributions to other people, then you'll answer in the affirmative. There is another altruistic reason why you should get this kind of work done if you need it.

A mentor once told me, "If you're trying to give to everybody else, but your own cart is empty, what are you going to give?"

You're responsible for filling yourself up so you have enough to give to others no matter if it's intellectually, mentally, emotionally, or spiritually.

For many, getting their smile back fills them up in a way that they never thought possible. It literally changes their life. It affects their work, their love life, and their relationships with friends and family.

But the biggest change is how they feel about themselves. I've had many a patient say, "I did this because it was my turn. I've been doing for others for so long; Now it's time for me."

And they're right. It was their turn. For me, this kind of dentistry is the most challenging and the most difficult. It also has the biggest rewards.

And as you've read, fixing a broken smile is about more than your looks. It's about your health. It's about how you're going to live your life. It is about recovering from the ravages of the past and finally getting the look you'd like to have.

Could it create a whole new you? It just might. We have seen it do the same for so many.

No dentist can guarantee that it'll change your life. But any of us can tell you this: smile transformations mean profound differences for many, and have changed many lives for the positive.

I remember one specific patient who got three promotions during the few months we were treating him. As he went from having unsightly gaps and holes in his mouth to actually having a full beautiful smile, he really blossomed. I'm not sure it was the smile that changed things so much for him or how much better he felt about himself.

Frustrations and Disappointments

We hear many patients express frustrations and disappointments to us. I'd like to address some of those here.

A common one is: I'm so embarrassed about my teeth that I was almost ashamed to open up to let you see.

We understand. We do this kind of work on a regular basis, so we understand how you feel. Rest assured, it would be nearly impossible for us to be shocked or surprised at anyone's condition. So just relax. We do this all the time.

We can help virtually everybody. Sometimes it takes a lot of work, a lot of time, a lot of money and many months of care, but we can help virtually anyone. Other times, few simple changes can make a profound difference.

The good news is you don't have to wait months and months to get a smile back. You could start on your own route back right away. Often we can improve things in just one or two visits while you are in treatment.

Another question that's not so much stated, as sensed: Who can I trust? I've tried dental care in the past. I've spent thousands and yet here I am again.

We understand. Usually it is impossible for us to know your circumstances and what went on in the past. What we can do is to ferret out why you are having problems now and give you measures to stop them in the future.

The biggest mistake you as a consumer can make is not making sure that you've had a complete diagnosis of the problem. While there may be one diagnosis, there are many ways to solve each problem.

It is our job to help you decide on the optimum way for you to fix your teeth and get healthy again. This can involve teeth that don't come out or removable teeth. The more you want your teeth to look, function and be like natural teeth, the higher the fee will be to get you there.

So, if you've been disappointed in prior care, there are generally three reasons. One, inadequate diagnosis of the problems and their root causes. Two, you didn't complete the care recommended, or three,

In dentistry we're working with you on three levels.

- **Prevention:** prevent problems in the first place. This requires at least two visits a year for maintenance and procedures that prevent problems of cavities, gum disease, and bite problems in the first place

- **Solving the problems:** We're solving the problems with you; working together to manage your experience comfortably.

- **Prevention and maintenance again.** Ensuring the treatment that has been done continues to work well and preventing new problems.

it was an inadequate plan of care for what you wanted and needed.

Now, it can be hard for you to know these things. So, in evaluating a dentist you want to make sure that they can show you before and after pictures of cases they have done. Make sure they can show you pictures of the same types of cases as yours, with the same solutions. Check for testimonials from patients, and see what other dentists say about them. Take a close look at their schooling, ongoing training, and if possible, what their staff thinks of them.

All of these can help you decide if you've found the right place. Just because someone has years and years of experience does not mean that they are qualified to help you. Excelling at this kind of dentistry is all about talent, training, care, skill, experience and judgment.

"Why didn't anyone tell me about all my problems before?" People ask me that a lot.

Well, it is possible that someone did try to tell you before but you weren't open to hearing the story at that time.

Maybe the person working with you didn't know enough to tell you everything you need to know or was in some way inadequate in helping you arrive at an understanding of what needed to be done.

Lastly, it is possible they didn't check everything that needed to be checked. They weren't comprehensive in their evaluation of you.

A lament I hear is: "No matter what I do, nothing seems to work."

If that is true for you, there is a reason. It comes from what I call Scotch tape dentistry. That's dentistry that's a patch or short-term solution. The more complex your needs and problems, the more you need complete care to insure that it will work.

Another comment almost every dentist hears: "I didn't know my teeth affected my health."

As you've already read in this book, your teeth and gums matter to your health to a great extent. Their health does affect the quality of your life. So, there's no question about that any more.

Another comment I hear: The dentist didn't seem interested in me.

If you want any dentist to be interested in you, get interested in your own dental health and listen to what the dentist has to say. Get involved. Get interactive. Accept treatment suggestions rather than deny them.

It is important for a dentist to be interested in you. The dentist should listen to your concerns and answers your questions.

Unknowingly, some people will say things to a dentist like, "No hard feelings, doc, but I hate dentists," or "Nothing seems to work," and it's all negative, negative, negative, at some point even the very best dentists are going to say, "Gosh, I'm dealing with someone who won't even hear what I have to say. I can really help him if he will let me."

The reality is that a relationship with a dentist is very much like a health partnership. We have to work together to get your oral health in order and keep it that way. Without your cooperation, we can do little that matters to you, long term. This is quite unlike a physician's workings with you. A visit to your medical doctor is usually short and involves a brief exam and typically a prescription for a medication. We, as dentists, are performing procedures. Our time together is longer and we must have your cooperation and help to get the work done at all.

Another common frustration is the fact that fixing your teeth and your smile does cost a lot. There's no doubt. But it's worth every penny.

People have a natural tendency to forget something once it's fixed. Unfortunately, problems don't stay solved unless they're maintained. People who religiously change their oil every 3,000-5,000 miles, paint their house every five years, or clean their windows every spring, very often forget about their dental care.

The solution is to find a dentist you can trust and work with the doctor as a partner. Get your care done completely, while working together with your dentist to maintain your teeth and create a positive dental experience.

Consider the dentist's world. He spends his day doing meticulous procedures through a three inch hole, upside down and backwards in a mirror on a squirming patient. Most good dentists work with magnification optics and work to tolerances of tenths of millimeters, smaller than the period of the end of this sentence. Top dentists have highly developed hand-eye coordination and manual dexterity. Every filling or restoration done is a completely custom job.

When completed, every dental restoration is subjected to a harsh environment. It is under water and in acid and digestive enzymes 24/7. They are subject to hundreds of pounds of pressure a thousand times a day and go from hot coffee to freezing ice cream. It is nothing less than miraculous that dental restorations exposed to these factors can last 10-15-20-30 or more years. If someone built a car or a watch or a house that lasted that long under these conditions they would be on the cover of Time Magazine....perhaps win a Nobel Prize.

Cindy's Story

When Cindy came in she quickly told us why. "I want a beautiful smile again," she related while we did our patient interview.

Cindy had been divorced for six months, after years of a marriage that had been rocky.

"It's time to focus on me," was her comment as to why she was getting this done now. "Besides, my ex-husband is paying for it... and he should after all those years I gave him."

While she never quite said it, we got that Cindy's prior husband had left her for a younger woman. (That was later confessed.)

Cindy showed us a picture of herself smiling from her college yearbook at Duke. "Can you make my smile look like that again?" she almost pleaded.

Now whenever a person gives a picture that shows how her smile looked from twenty five years ago, I pause. Here is the surprise-the answer can often be yes. However, the other factors of the face, lips and aging signs show effects too. We can't always duplicate that smile, but still, we can make it look sooo much better that our patients are elated.

For Cindy, her knockout, good looking smile was possible again based on our complete dental physical.

Admittedly, the work was extensive. We had to integrate multiple types of procedures working with gum repositioning, tooth symmetry, tooth position, implants, root canals, etc. In other words, it took all of our skills and training and experience. Often these procedures had to be done together at one longer appointment.

Cindy was anxious to look good again as soon as possible. While it can take many months to get totally finished, we can have a patient's smile looking good again usually within the first couple of visits.

When we completed Cindy's smile makeover, we handed her a mirror. Tears welled up in her eyes.

"I'm so happy. My smile looks great," she gushed. Now the tears were flowing pretty good. Often the emotional angst has been pent up so long that when the smile relief comes, tears flow. Tears of joy. That is one of those moments of enormous psychic payback for a dentist like me. All those years of training and toiling to be the best we can be are all pointed to making a difference in people's lives. People like Cindy.

We took pictures of her new smile. She insisted on pictures with us in them, too.

We have kept up with Cindy through her regular maintenance check-ups that we insist patients have. It makes no sense to get all that beautiful work done and then not take care of it.

Cindy had jumped back into the dating game. About a year after we had completed her smile rejuvenation, Cindy came strutting in holding up her left hand. She was sporting a rock so big that a bragging rights certificate comes with it.

"I'm engaged!" she squealed. Our whole team congratulated her. We felt so happy for her. We love to see our patients doing well in life.

Cindy told us about meeting him. She was in a local upscale department store. He had noticed her beaming smile from across the room.

"He followed me to the coffee shop and struck up a conversation. I was so excited. I mean this guy was a hunk. He told me that my smile was the magnet that drew him in."

Now Cindy's new husband is a patient of ours too.

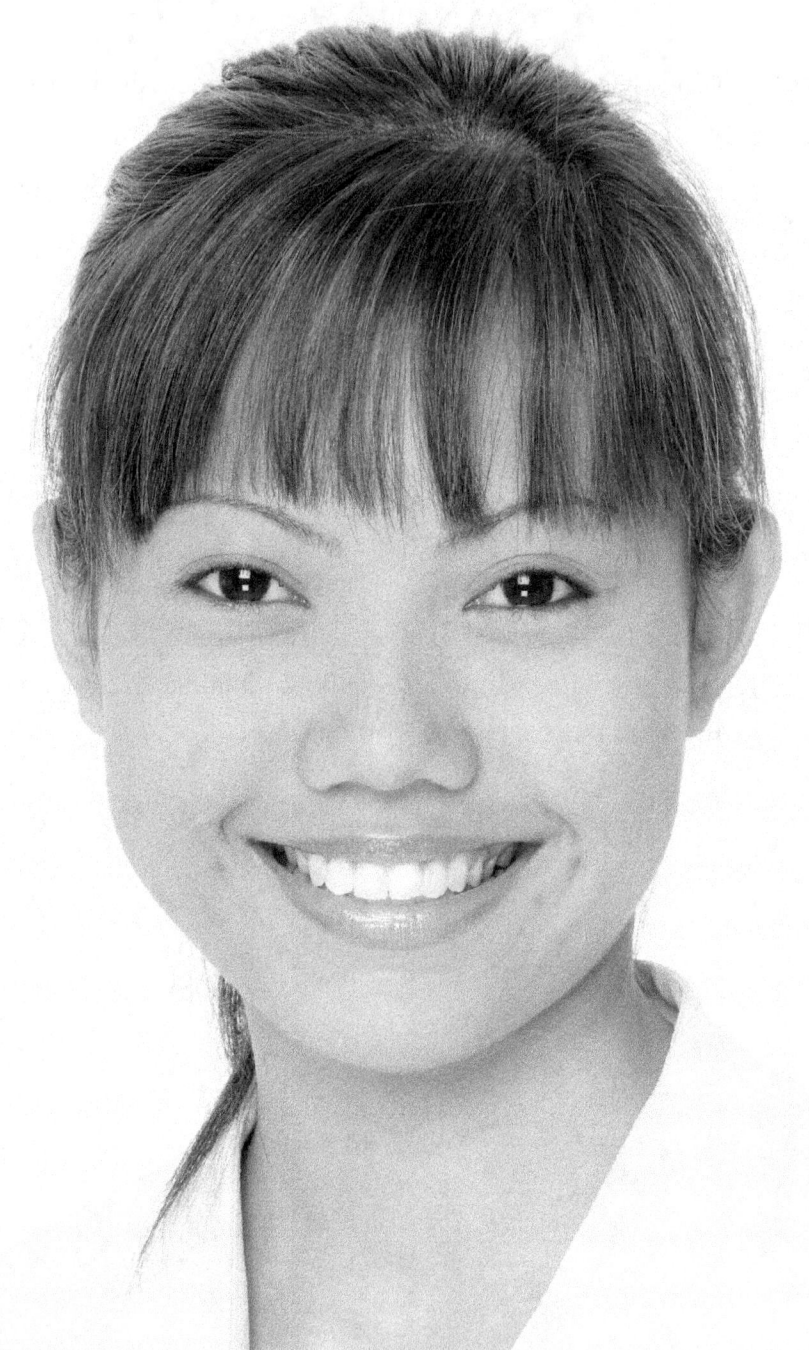

Gum Disease

CHAPTER 8

Gum Disease (Periodontitis)

Gum disease, also known as periodontal disease or periodontitis, is something that has been with man for thousands of years. Early man didn't experience gum disease seriously enough for it to be written about or talked about except in some ancient Indian texts. The reason is that the average life span was quite short, around age 21 at the time of Alexander the Great. Periodontitis simply did not have the time to develop.

As life spans got longer over time, gum disease became more prevalent.

As man is living longer, the need to keep your teeth in good health grows, too. Understanding gum disease and its effects is very important to your life and health.

Even in societies that had no refined sugar, gum disease was still prevalent. This has been found through anthropological digs that showed gum disease around the teeth on skulls.

So, what's this got to do with you? A lot. Gum disease is one of the leading causes of tooth loss, and it affects your entire body and overall health.

When gum disease is present, treating it and stopping it takes time, energy and effort on your part and on your dentist's part. Not treating it is worse, far worse.

In fact, if you have gum disease you should think of it as a chronic problem that you'll have to manage the rest of your life. To think otherwise is kidding your self. This proactive approach yields the best long-term results.

If you had gum disease and "It went away," then you're four times more likely to get it again than someone who never had gum disease in the first place.

So, why is it so wicked? What's so difficult about gum disease? The effects of periodontal disease are silent at first, no pain and no outward signs of trouble except for a little gum bleeding when you brush. From there, gum disease can progress rapidly, sometimes taking only weeks to cause major destruction. However, it most often takes longer to wreak its havoc. Over a period of time, the gum disease gets worse and more clinical signs can be picked up by your dentist. You'll start to notice more bleeding, teeth that get loose and bad breath that won't go away. At the terminal stages, overt pain starts to be felt. Bone and supporting gum tissue have been lost. Now you can visually see it!

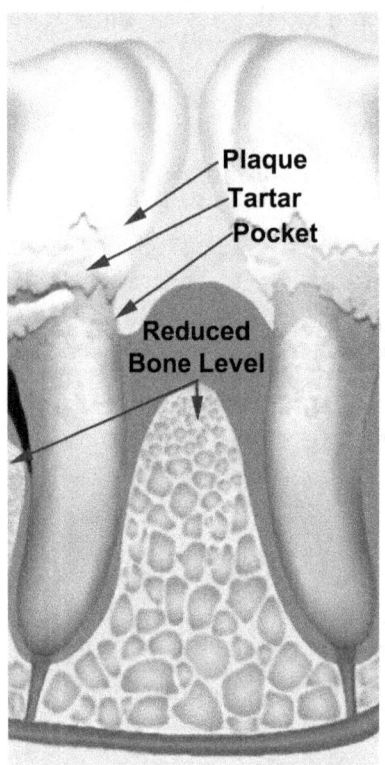

Plaque
Tartar
Pocket

Reduced
Bone Level

When you can see it, you are already in big trouble. When pain increases – and it will for most – the trouble means teeth need to come out. The lack of pain lulls people into thinking "it is just a little problem" or "it will get better on its own," or "I am fine. My gums just bleed and they do that all the time so it must be normal." This is wishful thinking. People who believe this are kidding themselves to the detriment of their own health and the family and friends who love them.

What people don't know is that the bacteria that cause gum diseases can be passed from one human to another, especially those that live together, sharing food and drinks.

So how does this get started? It starts with a biofilm called plaque.

What is dental plaque? Bacteria live in and around your mouth just like they do throughout your digestive tract. That's normal.

Dental plaque is a sticky, nearly invisible substance that adheres to the teeth, the gums and the tooth roots. It is a biofilm created by these oral bacteria. These bacteria secrete acids and enzymes that cause inflammation in the tissue and breakdown of the bone. Moreover, these bacteria stimulate an immune response from your body when the biofilm has been on a tooth long enough that actually causes bone to melt away. Your body "sees" the bacteria as disease and starts a chain of events to shed this diseased tooth and tissue away from the body.

There are different stages of gum disease. The first one is called gingivitis. Gingivitis quite literally means "inflammation of the gingiva" or gum tissue around the teeth. Gingivitis is reversible. It is confined to the soft tissue. If left untreated, it can progress into increasingly severe levels of periodontitis, permanent loss of gum attachment and bone.

Perio- means "around" and *dont-* means "tooth": The tissues around the tooth. With periodontitis, bacteria attack the tiny little ligaments that hold teeth in place next to bone, embed themselves into the outer layers of the tooth root and then infiltrate the bone itself.

Then these bacteria infiltrate into the gum tissues and often end up circulating throughout the entire body. In fact, cultures have found oral bacteria in the arterial plaques in the blood vessels in coronary arteries.

There are bacteria that we consider "good ones" and some we consider "bad ones." Here's how it usually develops.

These bad bugs **evolve over time**. Studies have shown that bacteria evolve from good ones to bad ones over a period of about 13 *weeks*, assuming that the bacteria contained in dental plaque are not cleaned off. They evolve over this short period of weeks from benign oxygen loving ones to destructive anaerobic ones that can thrive deep in the little pocket next to your tooth. Anywhere in your mouth that you can't, don't or won't clean thoroughly is subject to gum disease.

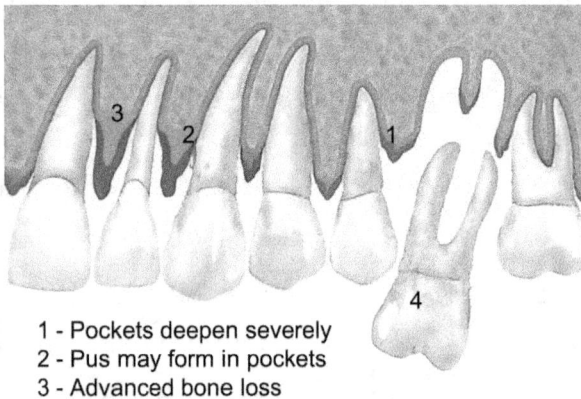

1 - Pockets deepen severely
2 - Pus may form in pockets
3 - Advanced bone loss
4 - Teeth become very loose, and may
 fall out or need to be extracted

Severe Periodontitis

Over time, the normal healthy environment around the teeth degrades. Without daily removal with brushing and flossing, the bacteria find protection by invading deeper into the tissues. The deeper they are able to invade, the harder it is for you to mechanically remove them. Once the damage is done, the bacteria are able to go where your toothbrush and floss can't reach! These bacteria that adhere to your teeth lie deep down inside pockets next to your tooth roots have a lovely environment. They've got warmth, they have shelter inside those pockets, and

Biofilm Plaque Formation

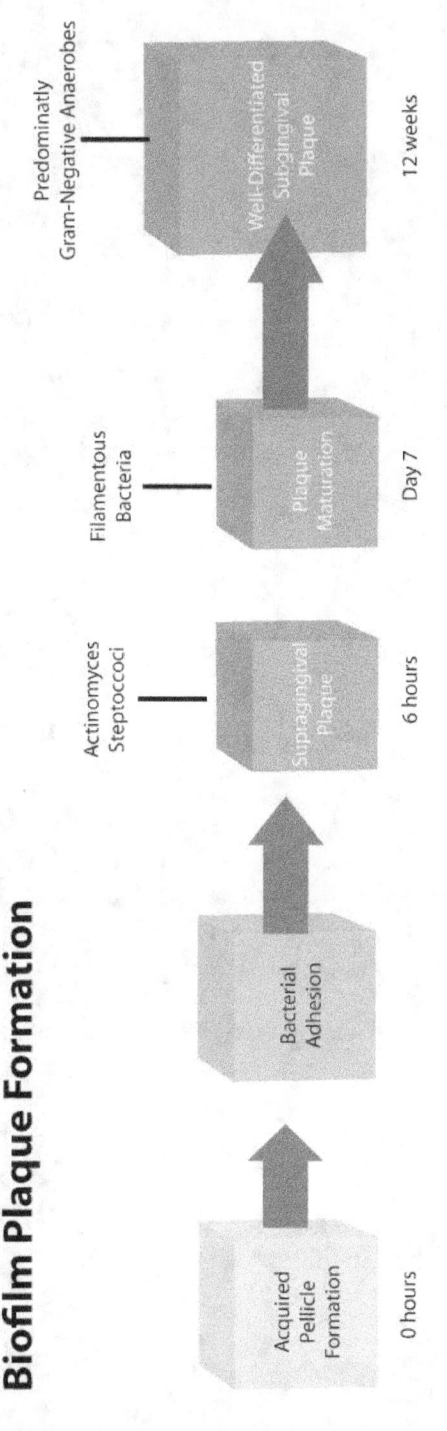

Acquired Pellicle Formation — 0 hours

Bacterial Adhesion

Supragingival Plaque — 6 hours
Actinomyces
Steptoccoci

Plaque Maturation — Day 7
Filamentous Bacteria

Well-Differentiated Subgingival Plaque — 12 weeks
Predominatly Gram-Negative Anaerobes

Cycle of Plaque

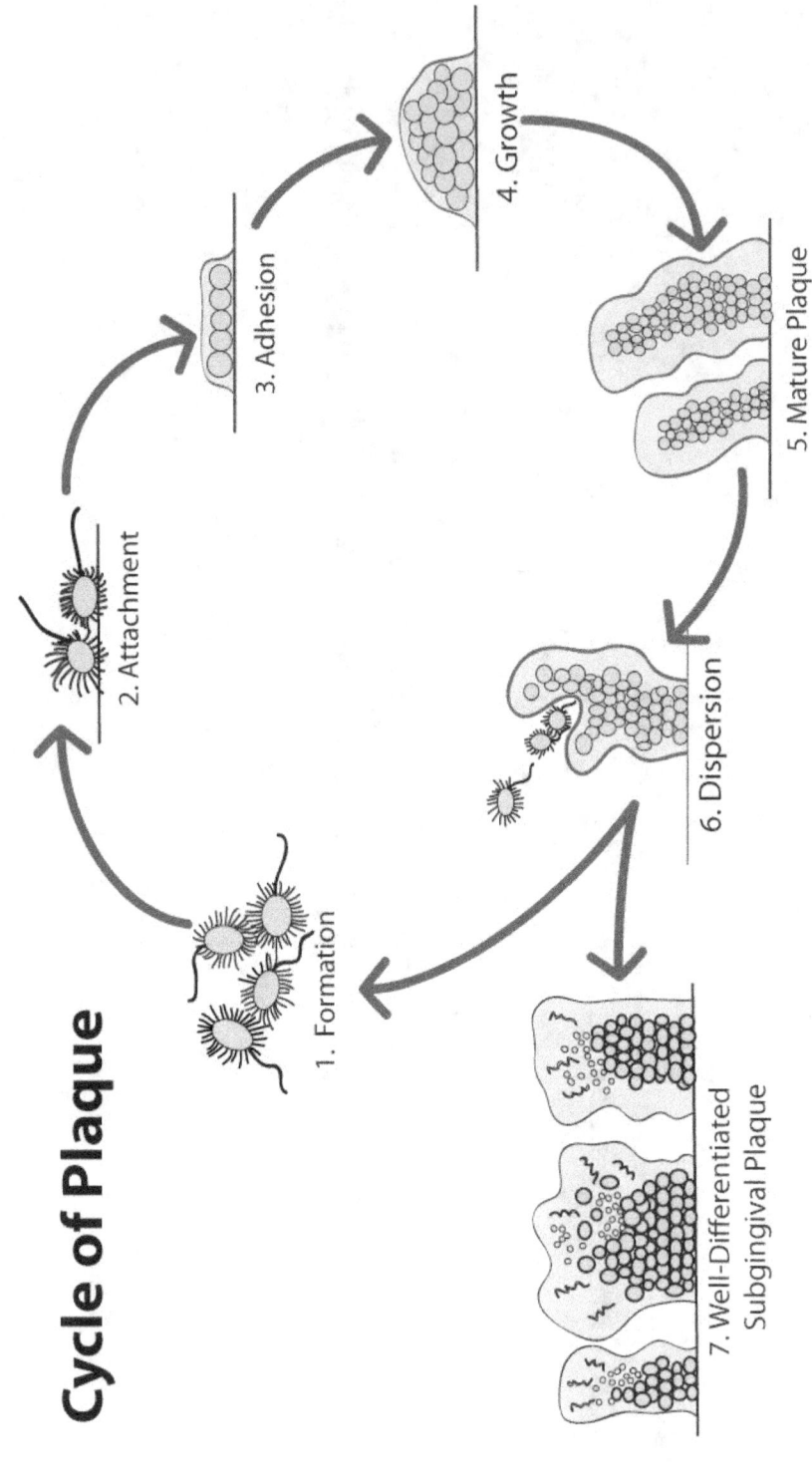

1. Formation
2. Attachment
3. Adhesion
4. Growth
5. Mature Plaque
6. Dispersion
7. Well-Differentiated Subgingival Plaque

they've got a food source: the foods you eat. And as you might guess, the more sugar you give them, the happier they are.

What's frightening is that these single-celled bugs evolve to act like multi-cellular organisms. Over time they evolve and actually reach out to other bacteria and connect with one another. Now instead of acting like single cell bacteria, they become almost like multi-cellular organisms, capable of acting together to survive your attempts to eradicate them. In response to your cleaning efforts and your body's immune system, they can change their shape, secret protective layers to hide under, and secrete enzymes to inactivate the body's defenses. Meanwhile, they are fighting for their survival and secreting toxins and enzymes into the gum tissue.

These periodontal pathogens can make themselves almost hidden to your immune system by inactivating the antibodies your body sends to fight them. It is like the bacteria have kryptonite to fight the Superman antibodies your body sends out to rescue your gums. Then, comes the scary part. The teeming bacteria will cause an immune response that causes the body itself to remove the bone around the diseased teeth so the teeth can come out. The body decides that if it can't overcome the bacteria, it will remove the body parts that are holding on to them. It is as if the body itself is amputating the disease laden tissue rejecting the teeth.

These pathogens cause ulcerations inside the gum tissue where you can't see. To get an idea of the size of this ulcer, look at the palm of your hand. In cases where the gum bleeds around virtually every tooth, the *ulcerated tissue could be as large as the size of the palm of your hand*. These bacteria infiltrate into the body through the blood stream increasing inflammation and sapping the body's energy and ability to handle stress. Research continues to find more and more diseases and health conditions affected by periodontal disease. The list is long already and getting longer!

Everybody has this biofilm we call plaque. To maintain dental health you must mechanically remove the dental plaque from your teeth and tooth roots. That means physically scraping with a toothbrush or dental floss - something to mechanically remove it. Washing it away won't work. Mouthwash won't work. They help you feel better but fail to remove the biofilm. That biofilm is one tough cookie.

Here are some of the areas of study of periodontitis and the effects on you:

- Coronary Artery Disease-A British study showed that poor oral hygiene and periodontitis both increased the risk of coronary heart disease by 25 percent.
- In that same study, the risk was 72 percent higher among younger men under the age of 50.
- Heart Attack - Researchers determined that people who have markers for periodontal disease in their bloodstream ran a **risk of heart attack that was two to four times higher than those who didn't have periodontitis.**
- The American Heart Association has identified periodontitis as one of the major chronic infections that put you at higher risk for atherosclerosis and coronary heart disease later in life.
- Pregnancy Risks – increased incidence of low birth weight babies, premature births and preeclampsia (dangerous high blood pressure) during pregnancy
- Increased Lung problems – affecting pneumonia, emphysema and other respiratory problems
- Diabetes – worsened by periodontitis and vice versa
- Stroke – gum disease can double the risk
- Cancer – increased incidence of cancer
- Arthritis – increased severity of rheumatoid arthritis and osteoarthritis

---

Active Treatment – not Watch and Wait – While Periodontal Disease is at hand

For many people with periodontal disease they *must see a dentist for active care* to a.) get these bacteria cleaned out and b.) to enable the tissues to heal so the area become cleansable again. Without active treatment from a dentist who understands this process, you are doomed to lose some or all of your teeth.

Eighty-five percent of the problems occur between teeth where your brush can't reach. That is why dentists prescribe dental floss use. Floss isn't the only way to get between teeth, we have others.

By the way, this thirteen week period of bacterial evolvement into destructive bacteria is the reason for returning to your dentist every 3 months for maintenance. If you have had gum disease, these every 13 week periodontal therapy sessions wipe out the bad bugs and start the cycle all over again.

I suggest if you are a non-flossing person that you request your dentist to show you other ways to clean between your teeth.

When these bacteria have remained on the teeth and roots for weeks, months and years, their destructiveness multiplies – bad breath that won't go away; bone loss; spongy, red inflamed gums that bleed when you brush; loose teeth; pain and tooth loss are the typical results. Not a pretty picture. The stark truth is that it is even worse, as I'll describe later.

Not knowing the truth about your mouth gets you in trouble. That is one of the big reasons for this book – so you can know.

Even Shakespeare wrote about "being long in the tooth". That is as a result of gum disease causing a breakdown of bone and gum tissue around it.

Gum disease is serious for you. Not only can it become a serious reason for losing your teeth, more and more evidence leads one to realize that it can cause one to lose his life.

Gum disease causes an inflammatory chain reaction that affects your whole body.

One of the main precepts of current dental medicine is that oral infection causes a chronic inflammatory burden on the body's entire system. It's based in part on evidence that oral pathogens have evolved the capacity to directly invade tissues throughout the system, triggering inflammatory events that have consequences for other organs and systems.

Cancer

A study from the Harvard School of Public Health analyzed data from the Health Professionals Follow-up Study, which gathered health issue data from over 51,000 American men.

Their findings, released in 2007, showed that, after adjusting for age, smoking, diabetes, body mass index and other factors men who had periodontitis were *63 percent more likely to develop pancreatic cancer than those who did not have periodontitis*. Researchers also found that non-smokers who had periodontitis had a two-fold increase in the risk of pancreatic cancer as did those who did not have periodontitis.

 Find out more at http://www.hsph.harvard.edu/hpfs/hpfs_pubs2007.html

Another study, released in May 2008, indicates that men with a history of periodontitis had a 14% higher overall risk of cancer than those who didn't have periodontitis whether they were smokers or non-smokers.

There are other types of cancers related to periodontitis. Recent research published in the British medical journal *Lancet Oncology* found that people who had periodontitis also ran a **36 percent higher risk of lung cancer, even if they had never smoked**. If they had fewer teeth than normal, indicating serious periodontitis that resulted in tooth loss, their risk of lung cancer was **70 percent higher.** The risk of *kidney cancer was 40 percent greater.* Risks for blood cancers – such as non-Hodgkin lymphoma, leukemia and multiple myeloma – were **50 percent higher.**

Not surprisingly oral cancers are more likely to strike people with periodontitis, according to a University at Buffalo study released in 2003. One of the study co-authors, Dr. Sarah Grossi, noted that previous research had shown associations between other infections and cancer such as H. pylori and stomach cancer, the human papillomavirus, and cervical cancer.

So just how serious is periodontal disease? The implications are frightening, wouldn't you agree?

When people say, "I don't want to have gum treatment or gum surgery done," it's understandable. Most of the surgery in the past was all reductive in nature and involved cutting tissues away, exposing lots of tooth roots. There was a lack of knowledge about the disease that we have now. Today is different.

For example, as a result of DNA research we know there are some 800 different types of bacteria that live in your mouth in and around tooth roots. Not all of them are pathogenic or disease causing.

Gum Disease Treatment

You no longer have to deal with having spaces and exposed roots and sensitive teeth any longer. Now we're able to treat your gums conservatively. We're able to do additive surgery, as opposed to the reductive surgeries of the past. We can actually graft new bone in place. Or, if the tooth is too far gone, we'll take it out and place a modern implant.

So, the good news is gum disease can be defeated. But the other reality is that you have to do your part. It does some take time and effort, but it is worth the effort, isn't it?

Help to improve your oral home care

Most people should use a power toothbrush. A power toothbrush is assisted by a battery, that enables the bristles to move faster than you can make them move manually. The average person will manually create 300 strokes a minute. Many of these power-assisted toothbrushes run at 30,000 strokes a minute. Moreover, most people spend far too little time using a toothbrush. Most people spend about thirty seconds. You should take two minutes and systematically go throughout the mouth to ensure no area is missed. Most power toothbrushes have timers that allow you to know how long you have been brushing.

That's an enormous difference in cleaning ability between the manual and power-assisted brush. Simple math tells you that two minutes at 30,000 brush stroke a minute is better than 300 brush strokes for thirty seconds. So, for most people, particularly those with gum disease, having a power-assisted toothbrush is a *very* good idea. Thirty seconds isn't enough.

Times Have Changed

Dentists have a wide array of treatments for periodontal diseases. While treatment could be difficult in the past, times have changed as have our therapies. Today it is more effective, more comfortable, easier and better than ever before.

Gum disease treatment can include lasers, antibiotic therapies, immune system modifiers, antimicrobial solutions, and DNA testing. More than ever before we are better able to stop gum disease.

Difficult Periodontal Surgery Is Gone

Before the disease had gone on too long, we were forced into last gasp, hero-type periodontal surgery. We wanted to save your teeth because the alternative was worse. This was challenging, expensive and not always successful long term. Healing times could be extended and frankly, it could be pretty darn uncomfortable while healing.

Today, this type of periodontal surgical intervention has been largely displaced by the use of dental implants. Out with the bad tooth or teeth, and in with the man made, biologically compatible artificial tooth roots to re-build the missing teeth. Faster, easier, more predictable and more comfortable. There is an entire chapter dedicated to this subject later on that you want to be sure to read.

Gum disease no longer has to be the main cause of tooth loss. However, it can't be ignored.

Good news. We can conquer gum disease. A second piece of good news: if you have a tooth that's so far gone that you can't bring it back to health with conventional gum therapy, either reductive or additive, we can now place dental implants to replace those missing teeth.

The worst thing you can do is to hold on to teeth that should have come out long ago.

I'll tell you why it's bad. If you're holding on to a tooth because you don't want to lose it but you know you've got gum disease around it, here's what will happen.

The body will remove the bone that surrounds the tooth for you. In such instances, people can remove teeth by taking their fingers and wiggling it out.

The worst part, is that the body destroys the bone that could've been used for placing dental implants. So, it makes your care more challenging, more difficult and more expensive.

So, if you have gum disease, get it treated. If you're going to lose a tooth because of gum disease get it taken out without delay.

Gum disease does not have to be something that ruins your smile. It can be treated. It can be handled. But you've got to act and take care of it.

With the antibiotics that we presently use, the techniques we presently use, the type of surgery that we presently use, gum disease does not have to get the best of you.

Kathy's Story

Colorful. Some might say outlandish. I say good for them. When Kathy came in she was wearing a purple dress with red accessories and a feathered hat. Her hat looked like something out of a movie. Large, ostentatious, a statement maker. What did it say?!

This was my first introduction to the Red Hat Society. My new patient, Kathy, was quick to explain her unusual garb. She told me it was a social group of ladies that started in the late 90's that just took off. Now there are hundreds of chapters all over.

I asked her what they did. The answer was quick. "We meet, eat, talk and travel. Our mission is to enjoy our lives and add a bit of flair. Thus the red and purple colors."

I liked her immediately.

"Kathy, how did you find us?" I inquired.

"I was referred by one of your patients, my friend and fellow Red Hat member, Helen. I want you to help me have a smile like hers."

I smiled. Helen was a terrific gal. She had started as a reluctant patient who wanted to do as little as possible until we explained the good common sense reasons for getting her smiled really fixed. Helen, once she discovered the value, had become a big advocate for our special level of dentistry: it makes you look good, feel good, chew better and the dentistry lasts. Plus, it makes for a happier, healthier you.

Helen's enthusiasm (after all, she was a Red Hat lady) had rubbed off on Kathy.

Still, Kathy had some concerns and reservations. Virtually everyone does. She was concerned about being comfortable before and after treatment, concerned about the dollars involved and how much needed to be done. All normal.

Honestly, Kathy's mouth just didn't match the rest of her. Her teeth made her look older. She had lost some teeth that had caused her bite to start collapsing and her front teeth to shift, twist and turn. The years of her admitted neglect had taken its toll.

It makes no sense to chastise patients for errors of the past. Finger wagging and "you are so wrong" lectures are forbidden in my office. My feeling is that "Hey, the patient is here. Let's move forward without criticizing and demeaning the person in my chair who came here for help." Wouldn't you agree?

We performed our complete dental physical as she needed far more than just a regular checkup. What we found was both challenging and heartening. Kathy was going to need to lose some very bad teeth. Not only was I concerned about what the really bad ones were doing to her mouth, but also to her overall health. Kathy was diabetic so she couldn't afford the repercussions of such a badly diseased mouth.

That's another thing. Kathy, like so many others, knew her teeth looked bad and she knew she had a bad taste in her mouth. She had just never realized how important oral health was to her total body health.

At her consultation, Kathy was surprised at first by the investment involved. That's typical. It is not unusual for these types of cases to be in the low to high tens of thousands.

Once we explained what we were doing and why, we showed her the smile we had created for her with our computerized technology.

Her first question after we showed it: "You can make my teeth look like that?"

We assured her that we could. In fact, most often, the final result is better than the computer simulation. (We do these simulated after pictures before you start so you can see what you'll be getting. This is also why we ask patients to bring in pictures of themselves or others smiling, showing us how they want to look. This way we can alter color, brightness, contour, size, texture and positioning so it fits your smile goal.)

"How soon can you start?" was her next question.

Today Kathy sports her beautiful big smile wherever she goes and particularly with her Red Hat Society tea parties. One of the society chapter members who didn't know her playfully accused her of being too young to be a member and insisted that Kathy take off her red hat and don the pink one of those less than 50 years old.

That made Kathy's day. And yes, she does look ten years younger today.

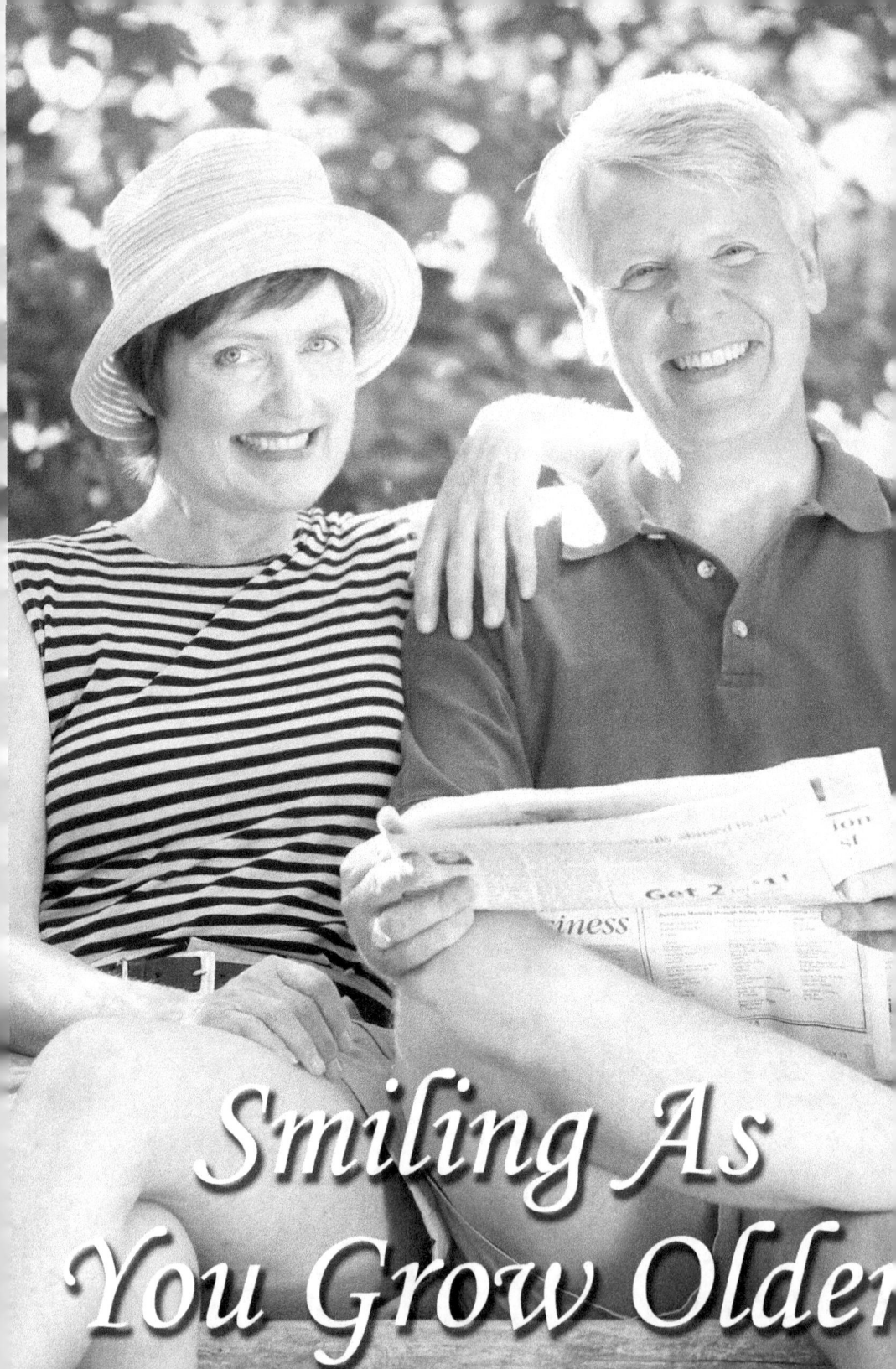

Smiling As
You Grow Older

CHAPTER 9
Smiling As We Grow Older

As we grow older our faces change. Gravity takes over. Between age 30 and age 70, we all experience significant facial changes that occur naturally because of gravity.

Your upper lip gets longer. Your lower lip gets more flaccid. You start to show less upper teeth, but more of your lower teeth.

As we age, we get wrinkles. Our face starts to show the crow's feet at the eyes and laugh lines around the face. We can get brown spots. Our skin can lose some of its elasticity. All of these combined can amplify each other.

Your smile can further amplify these aging effects or make them seem negligible. Often those who've had teeth removed but not sufficiently replaced, get more wrinkles. A lot more wrinkles. They look older – far older than their natural age.

I've seen many patients come to my practice who tell me that they're 55-years-old. A lot of these folks *look like they're 75-years-old!* I feel bad for them.

Many times they've come because they know they're in trouble.

Often they've put off dental care and the situation is now more than serious. It is dire. (We can still help change things dramatically for the good.)

Losing teeth can accelerate your aging. Loss of teeth without proper replacement can dramatically change the way you look. The changes in diet due to impaired or altered chewing ability further advance the aging process, often *making one look ten to twenty years older* than actual age.

You might be surprised at one of the main culprits that accelerates aging – the back teeth – also known as the molar teeth.

The molar teeth do the majority of your chewing. Many people end up losing their molar teeth when they're younger and never have them replaced. While the teeth themselves may no longer bother you, the adjacent teeth begin a silent migration, moving into angled positions that promote gum disease, decay and bite problems. All of this comes without pain – at first. The lack of symptoms can con you into thinking everything is OK. Just because you don't feel any symptoms does not mean that your dentist can't see any signs of problems. The dentist usually will.

When you try to chew without molar teeth, it means you have to chew on your front teeth. Front teeth were not designed by Mother Nature to function as grinding teeth. They were designed to function more like the way a pair of scissors works. That is, to cut. Front teeth take the first bite out of something and smile, all the rest of the work of chewing goes to the back teeth.

This is a very different function than grinding. Think of it like this: what happens to a pair of scissors you use to grind up anything? The edges are ruined. The same thing can happen to your front teeth when you have insufficient back teeth for chewing. Counting on your front teeth for chewing and grinding your food causes them to wear out far faster and can completely change your smile. You need back teeth to preserve the shape and good looks of your front teeth. Few people know that losing one's back teeth can cause the front teeth to wear out before their time. Now you do.

The Smile-Dominant Face

The good news comes in the form of the "smile-dominant" face. The smile dominant-face consists of a smile that is so big, bright and beautiful that it often makes facial wrinkles and blemishes fade into insignificance.

The smile-dominant face looks younger. It looks healthier, more vibrant.

A patient of mine recently said, "This is better than plastic surgery."

By creating a smile-dominant face we're able to take the emphasis off of the skin, wrinkles and blemishes that come with aging and deliberately place even more emphasis onto the teeth and smile. And when you have a great smile, you want to show it off, right?

On the other hand...

Do you hide your smile?

Many folks do hide their smiles. What does hiding your smile do to other people that look at you? They look at what's presented to them. They look at the skin. They look at the wrinkles, blemishes, lines and spots.

The smile-dominant face focuses people you meet away from the blemishes, wrinkles and signs of aging onto your gorgeous smile. That's where they normally want to go anyway. Wouldn't you rather have that, too?

Living Longer, Living Better

When you keep your teeth healthy and restore them to health, function and beauty and keep them that way, you very well may live longer.

This has been known empirically through our experience for many years as dentists. It's now being proven by science.

I run into a lot of aging people who don't restore and maintain their teeth because they assume they won't need them. After all, they are getting older. We are mortals after all. They don't think they will be around to use them, so why invest in their dental health?

This is <u>mistaken thinking</u> that simply comes from not knowing any better.

One problem with planning for the obsolescence of your teeth based on aging is that it often becomes a **self-fulfilling prophecy**. By simply not having your teeth, you're more likely to have a shortened life span simply because of poor nutrition and an altered ability to fight off disease and disability.

Another problem is the undesirable situation in which you outlive your teeth. This means a lessened quality of life *at the very time* where quality of life is most important to you.

Guessing how long you will live to determine whether or not to get your teeth in the best shape possible is a very big gamble that threatens you later on in life and robs your loved ones of the *experience of you*. Who wants to leave a legacy of toothlessness? Who wants to shorten their years needlessly? Your family and friends want you around to share in their lives.

Longer Life Spans

People are living longer. The speed with which longevity gains are being made is higher than it has ever been and increasing. In my opinion, people will, at some point, often live to see 120 years. How soon? I don't know. But with the total amount of science and data doubling every five years, I expect we'll see a steady increase in man's longevity. Research on aging continues as society demands it.

So if we're living longer, we need our teeth longer. Makes sense, right!

Interestingly, healthy, natural teeth could last up to a 150 year lifespan. So, that should give us some hint about what's possible.

You probably don't think about it, but how you look and interact with your children and grandchildren is part of the real legacy that you leave for them. Part of your **legacy** is how the people you love and who love you remember you.

Quite frankly, your smile can help you leave a legacy of cheer, love and joy. When your family thinks of you, they can think of you as having that great gorgeous smile and a happy demeanor. That legacy can be a difference maker far into the future.

More than one grandparent has told me of an incident where a grandchild has made a comment like, "How come you can take your teeth in and out, grandma?" Obviously, no parent or grandparent wants her child to think less of her because she is toothless. For many, this has been the deciding factor in the getting their teeth fixed.

Worn Out Dentistry

A lot of the folks in the boomer age group, all 78 million of them, have old dentistry that has worn out. If you have dental work that is fifteen, twenty, twenty-five years old, you are going to need to have more work done. Don't kid yourself into thinking it won't happen to you. It happens to everyone. It is just a matter of time. Old dark, stained or worn fillings **will** need replacement. The larger and older the restorations, the more critical it is to be proactive in replacement. Leaving failing dentistry in place threatens the health of the teeth by increasing the likelihood of decay or infection into the nerve within the tooth.

How do you know if the aging dentistry situation has happened to you? It starts with teeth becoming sensitive, stained, darker or worn. Often the teeth will have gum recession, causing teeth to look longer. Sometimes the old amalgam fillings are expanding silently, pulling away from the tooth structure, causing bacteria to leak into the teeth. Often, old fillings' expansion will break teeth and needlessly cause pain and an increase in treatment needed, requiring a root canal or extraction. Much of this could be avoided by replacing worn out restorations before this happens to you. Doesn't it make sense to prevent pain and increased dental expenses? You should check with your dentist to see when the right time is to replace old dentistry.

As you get older, you're going to have to get new work done to restore the work done years ago to help you preserve your teeth. If you don't, you could lose your teeth and the advantages of keeping them.

Living Differently Than Our Parents

Boomers aren't going to go gently into the night. Most want to lead full lives. Many are starting second careers. Some are returning to school. No one sees himself or herself in the human warehouse that so many nursing homes have become. Who wants to become a burden on their loved ones? That just isn't in your picture, right? Well, it could be in your future if you don't actively work with a knowledgeable, experienced dentist to keep your dental health at its best.

Boomers don't want to sit on a porch in a rocking chair, chomping their dentures together.

Healthy teeth can play a major role in giving you that quality and quantity of living that you'd like to have. If you can't eat right, the quality of your life diminishes along with your health.

Besides, eating what you want comfortably is one of life's true pleasures, wouldn't you agree?

Doris' Story

For Doris, losing her teeth and getting dentures at age 52 had been an unhappy choice she confided in us.

"At the time, I thought it was the least worst decision I could make. I had had trouble with my teeth for my entire life. I was glad to be rid of them. After I got my dentures, I thought I was doing OK with them. It was true that I had to focus a lot of attention on my false teeth. I couldn't eat what I wanted all the time. And after being re-fitted with new ones, my chewing was easier, but it wasn't long until my bones had shrunk more and once again I experienced insecurity about being out in public. I really hated that. It felt so confining.

"I had heard about dental implants, but thought they were going to be too expensive, so I just tried to get along with my dentures.

"One weekend, I was keeping my little treasure, my three year old granddaughter, Tiffany. Sometimes blessings come from unusual places. She watched me putting in my dentures. I could see her eyes get big. She said, 'Granny, why do you have teeth that you put in?' I was crushed. I didn't want this little light of my life thinking about me in any way like that. Plus, I knew I wasn't eating like I should. That's when I decided to call you."

After an examination and complete dental physical, we came up with a plan for Doris. We placed dental implants and made teeth for her that didn't come out. Doris loves her new smile and the comfort of knowing she wouldn't have any embarrassing denture moments ever again.

We knew what Doris wanted even if she couldn't, wouldn't and didn't know how to say what it was.

"When I am gone, I want her and all my grandchildren to remember me as the loving, smiling, kind grandmother – not as the unsmiling woman who took her teeth in and out.

"I am sooooo glad I had this done and I feel better about me. I feel more energized than before. And I am enjoying my food better than I have in years."

Removable
Teeth

CHAPTER 10
Removable Teeth
Dentures and Partial Dentures

Man is the only animal that can continue living without its teeth. Take the teeth away from any other animal and it dies.

Take the teeth away from man and there are choices. For some, removable teeth are the only solution. Others choose the better, more permanent solution afforded by today's technology.

In many respects, dentures are like oral wigs. Like a toupee or wig, they are but pale versions of the original, and most don't look very good.

Dentures are like that, too. They sit on top of your gums. *Some* can look pretty good. Most don't.

But because they're sitting on top of your gums, the force of chewing goes through the dentures to the soft tissue and bone underneath. Frequently, the soft tissue under a full or partial denture develops painful sore spots. The compression on the bone caused by the chewing on dentures inevitably leads to loss of bone. It is but a matter of time.

This loss of bone occurs in both height and width. This bone loss of the upper and lower jaws over time leads to wrinkles and for many, facial disfigurement.

Bone loss itself makes dentures more difficult to wear over time. There is just less to hold onto. I feel very sorry for the people in their 60's, 70's or 80's, who see dentures as the only solution to their problem. Why? Because their ability to accommodate new dentures is decreased just because of their age.

As we grow older, our capacity for accommodation decreases. We see that on all sorts of levels. We see it in our athletic ability. We see it in our stamina. It should not be a shock or a surprise that our ability to accommodate dentures decreases as we grow older.

Many dentures are made slap-dash for economic reasons. Some people don't know that there are other options. There are. If dentures are not custom made to fit the face, personality and chewing mechanism, people are often quick to develop that "denture look." Worse, poorly fitting dentures worsen bone loss all by themselves. This loss of bone further worsens the fit which further worsens the bone loss. This continues in a dwindling spiral with the denture wearer the biggest loser.

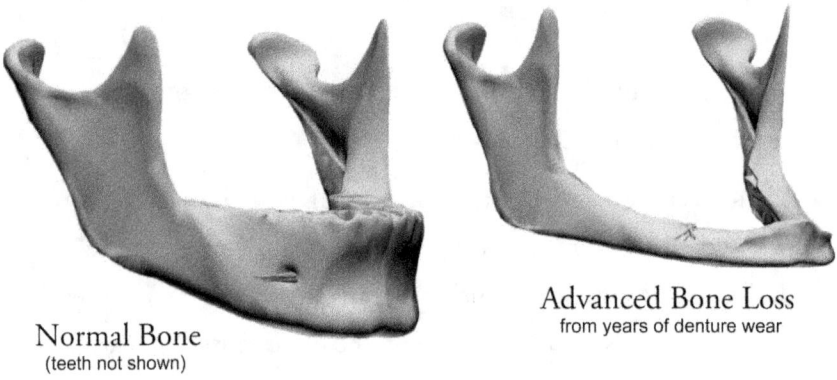

Normal Bone
(teeth not shown)

Advanced Bone Loss
from years of denture wear

The average denture wearer should have his denture relined or remade within one year of first receiving them. After three years, another reline is probably necessary. After seven years, a new set is needed. Few denture wearers adhere to a schedule of care like this at all. In fact, the average denture wearer goes to a dentist once every 14.9 years! There is a huge gap between what should be and what the public typically does. This failure to see a need for care makes the denture experience worse and puts the denture wearer at risk for increased oral cancer, especially for smokers.

Denture Adhesives

Denture adhesives have been around a long time. These are used to help stabilize dentures. In the U.S. alone, over 200 million dollars a year is spent buying this material. Evidently a lot of people want removable teeth that don't move around!

However, there is a problem. The greatest use of these glops, globs, powders and gels is to stabilize dentures that should have been re-made because of bone loss. Besides the taste, these adhesives leave a mess on one's mouth. I have seen patients come in with an immense wad of this stuff, trying to ring more use out of ill-fitting dentures. It is a big mistake.

The poorer the fit of the dentures, the greater the use of the goop to hold them in place. The poorer the fit, the greater the bone loss caused by the ill-fitting dentures! The very thing that is supposed to be helping is causing more loss of bone!

Is there ever a good use for a denture adhesive? Yes, there is. When a person wants the extra security that the adhesive gives them in public places, an adhesive can help out. No one wants to see a person's teeth fall out onto the plate in a restaurant. The real question is how much should be used? Just a tiny smidgen spread out over the whole denture. That is all that it should take to ratchet up the adherence to the tissues. It is so little that it is barely visible.

If the denture wearer is requiring more than just a little, then the likelihood is that the dentures should be replaced with better fitting ones.

What About Partial Dentures?

Given the choice between having no teeth or wearing a full denture, the partial denture can be a better choice. Why? Because a well-made partial denture distributes the bite force onto the remaining teeth as much as possible, away from the bone. This requires the partial denture to be rigid, usually made of metal and specifically made to use the teeth as anchors and retention of the partial denture.

Just as with the full denture, the gum and bone underneath the partial recede away. Mix in time and the loss of bone could be huge. A partial denture must be carefully planned and delivered so that the patient can function with them and bone is preserved as much as possible. The goal of a partial is to stabilize tooth positions and to provide chewing surfaces to chew against. It is not as good as chewing on healthy natural teeth.

Mistakes Patients Make With Partial Dentures?

- Failing to have good tooth support that takes pressure off the gums
- Failing to get a partial that is for more than just looks.
- Trying to use one's partials for something else
- Lack of supporting surfaces on teeth to stop an all plastic partial from digging into the gums.
- Failing to get a rigid partial made of metal that transmits bite force to the teeth.

Here is a real surprise: 40% of partial dentures stay in drawers, worn not at all or just for special occasions. Frequently, a person can chew better without the partial denture!

Like a full denture, if you must choose a partial, get one customized by a real expert to fit very well. It should distribute bite force over as large an area as possible to decrease force on bone. This also means it very well may need far more time effort and expertise to get one well made. The goal of a well made partial is to provide chewing surfaces, stabilize the remaining teeth's positions and minimize compressive force onto the bone. Remember that force on bone causes it to melt away over time.

Creating a well-made partial denture is a tall order. Even when done well, many people find partials too uncomfortable to wear. Many people consider the hooks of the partial denture fitting onto the remaining teeth to be so unsightly that they refuse to wear them.

Statistically speaking, teeth that anchor partial dentures are more likely to decay or get loose from the force put against them by the partial. If you are saying to yourself, "Why would anyone want a partial denture?" I understand. They should be avoided if possible.

What to Do If You Are Losing Your Teeth

Removable teeth are generally a poor solution for everyone. Avoid them if you can. And if you must lose your teeth consider how you could keep some tooth roots.

Why should you keep some tooth roots? If you can bring your tooth roots to an acceptable level of health, these can help preserve bone underneath a denture. Think of it as a way of cheating the denture demons.

Tooth roots stimulate bone to maintain itself. So, keeping tooth roots to go underneath a denture helps a person maintain their bone levels. Moreover, retaining tooth roots improves chewing function. Another advantage is the nerve endings around tooth roots give you a sense of spatial awareness. In other words, you have an increased awareness of "where your mouth is" when wearing this special variety of dentures

Dentures that fit over tooth roots are called overdentures, meaning that the dentures fit over the roots and come in and out just like regular dentures do. To use the overdenture techniques, your dentist must perform root canal treatment on the two to four teeth to be retained. Once these procedures are completed, the crowns of the teeth are cut off, leaving the roots at the gum level . The root canals done for this procedure are relatively easy for the patient to have done. What is so terrific about overdentures, particularly for the upper teeth, is that the roots preserve the bone and help the patient maintain his or her facial appearance. Overdentures are a real God-send when dental implants don't fit into a person's budget. Unlike the upper, the lowers are not good candidates for this procedure because the muscles of the cheek, lips and tongue displace a lower denture and make it move around during function. An upper denture can stay put pretty nicely because of the vacuum created between the overdenture and the upper jaw.

Keeping Bad Teeth Too Long

Sometimes, people hold on to bad, loose or diseased teeth for too long. This is a huge mistake. Why? Diseased teeth cause far more bone loss to occur faster than having the bad teeth

Wearing Dentures

The ugly truth is that many people with removable teeth never wear them. Many people, whether they have a full or partial denture, end up keeping their removable teeth in the nightstand drawer because they're so uncomfortable.

Dentures should be cleaned well daily and left out of the mouth a minimum of four hours a day. Dentures were never meant to be worn 24/7. Would you wear your shoes every minute of every day? No, you feet need to be rested. So do your gums underneath your dentures.

removed. More importantly, these infections from the bad teeth put your entire health at risk. Keeping bad teeth is a risk that just isn't worth taking.

Some denture wearers, having kept their teeth for too long, have lost so much bone that there is hardly any bone to support and retain a denture. In some of these cases, oral surgery must be performed to expose more jaw bone. Sadly, this complicates the dentist's work to use implants to rebuild the smile and chewing function. Often, there is not enough bone to anchor implants without doing bone grafting to rebuild the bone. Diseased, loose, failing teeth should be removed.

What to Do if You Already Have Dentures

For many people, dentures were the only option they had in the past when they lost their teeth. The reason, no matter what it was then, is now removed. Today you no longer have to wear dentures. The best option is to have dental implant treatment that protects and stimulates the bone to remain. This generally requires a number of implants sufficient to support the replacement teeth. Interestingly, the number of implants needed is dependent on the a person's age, bite function, total body size, density of bone and total bone volume. Everyone is different so there is no standard number to use. The number, type, and size of dental implants is based on diagnosis of your individual needs.

A mistake in getting dental implants is to use too few implants, thus the bone in the jaws continues to receive compressive force, melting it away. You wouldn't think that this would be a problem if the patient was receiving implant care, but using too few dental implants is commonplace among those dentists who are unaware of the real problem of bone loss. Any supposed economic advantage melts away also when too few dental implants cause an early demise to the replacement teeth.

Denture Reality

The more effort, expertise and talent that are brought to bear in making dentures, the better the fit, longevity and success of denture service. Even then, physiology is working against you and the dentist. Facial muscles, the tongue and bite pressures combine to make any denture difficult, and this is doubly so for the lower dentures.

It is no surprise when economy dentures fail. True, a few people can tolerate anything, but they are the rare exceptions, only a few out of a thousand patients can muster the energy to make quickie dentures really work – to tolerate them in spite of all the problems. Many a patient has been severely disappointed to learn about the inadequacies of these kinds of dentures through first-hand experience.

Making a set of dentures that are custom fit to match your level of bone, facial appearance, muscles, tongue and jaw movements is the best denture service investment.

The Importance of Your Bite

Did you know that ninety percent of sore spots under the removable teeth on the soft tissue are caused by a mismatched denture bite? It is true and too often, ignored except by the few dentists who have spent the time, money and effort to get the training to help those that wear dentures.

Recording the correct bite position in denture construction is a significant challenge. This is especially true for those who have lost significant bone already!

Clacking Dentures

You've probably been around someone whose dentures clack. It's embarrassing. They make noise all the time. Generally, that indicates one of two things.

The dentures are either too close together, or there's so little bone that the muscles in the floor of the mouth force the dentures up - making that clacking sound as the teeth of the upper and lower denture come together.

How Large Should A Denture Be?

You want a denture to be as large as possible and still go in the mouth. Why?

Because the larger the denture, the more that force is distributed over a larger area. The more the force is distributed over a larger area, the less compressive force against the bone, and therefore less bone is lost.

The problem with making dentures as large as possible is that muscle attachments get in the way, along with the tongue and the cheek. This problem is worse on the lower denture. Making an upper denture as large as possible can cause difficulties in swallowing and dislodge the upper denture.

So, it's always a balance between muscle position, tongue position, bite function and the amount of jawbone present to support the removable teeth. The longer one wears these removable dentures, the more damage is done to the bone that remains.

Force and Ability to Chew

Normal chewing force with natural teeth ranges from 25 pounds per square inch up to 75 pounds per square inch, with spikes going up to

250 pounds per square inch. Denture wearers experience progressive loss of chewing ability. The longer they are worn, the more difficult chewing can become. After a denture wearer has had dentures fifteen years or more, this chewing ability declines to about 5 pounds per square inch!

Final Recommendations

- If you must have dentures, get the best ones possible from an experienced dentist that makes high quality dentures on a regular basis. The dentist should make customized impressions, bite registrations and customized tooth arrangement. Often custom coloring of denture bases is needed to match the color of your gums.

- If you must have dentures, get upper overdentures if you can. These preserve bone better and protect your face better than full dentures.

- Replace your dentures every 7-8 years.

- Get relines every 2-4 years as needed to keep your dentures fitting as well as possible.

- Let your mouth rest at least 4 hours a day by removing your denture.

- If it is possible for you, get dental implants to avoid becoming toothless. If you are already a denture wearer, find a way to get dental implants. They can change your life.

As much as I've told you about dentures, understand this: any time that you can use dental implants or natural teeth in a healthy mouth instead of removable teeth, you're better off.

For some people, dentures are the only solution. In that case, get them made as well as you possibly can. But if possible, choose the alternative, dental implants.

Sarah's Story

Losing a tooth here and there hadn't seemed a big deal for Sarah.

"They were in the back. No one could really see they were missing. Or so I thought. It was at my niece's wedding reception that I heard the comment that shook me awake. I'll never forget it, 'Kim's Aunt Sarah looks so old compared to Kim's mom. Those missing teeth would make you think she is from the backwoods, a hillbilly or something.

"It was one of those bathroom conversations that were supposed to be private. I happened to be in there freshening up at the same time. I ran out with tears welling up in my eyes. I tried to forget about it and put on my social face. I couldn't stop thinking about those words. I excused myself and went to find a mirror where I could look at my face and smile privately. I found one and I took a good look. I didn't like what I saw. I wondered how many other people were saying to themselves what that young hussy had said!

"I am five years younger than Kim's mom, my sister, Lindsey. She looks like early 40's, late 30's!

"I started thinking about it, comparing Lindsey's smile to mine. I realized that I didn't look 50, I looked more like 60. My face had more wrinkles. My smile was dark, teeth were twisted and uneven.

"The mirror set I had found let me view my smile from the side. That's when I realized how much all those missing teeth showed and all the missing support for my face."

Lindsey sent Sarah to us. We were able to get her smile rejuvenation done by using dental implants, smile design and some newer therapies to regain lost bone. You should see her smile now. Sarah later told us, "It was a significant investment and it took more time and money that I thought it would. And I wish I had done something years ago. After you explained about my gum disease, I knew this wasn't just about my looks; it was about my health, too. I feel better now than I have in twenty years."

Sarah had a nasty case of gum disease that would have caused her to lose all her teeth had she delayed treatment any longer. Plus with what we now know about the mouth- body interactions and her family history of heart disease and cancer, Sarah's decision to get her smile back and teeth healthy again might just have saved her life. It was about 3 months after we had completed her extensive makeover with dental implants that we saw Sarah again for her now regular maintenance visit. The ring on her finger said it all. After being divorced for five years, she now had found the new love of her life. She smiled. She was beaming.

"Other people need to know about this. Most people don't know how important your smile and oral health is to your happiness and health," Sarah says.

We agree. That is one of the reasons for this book.

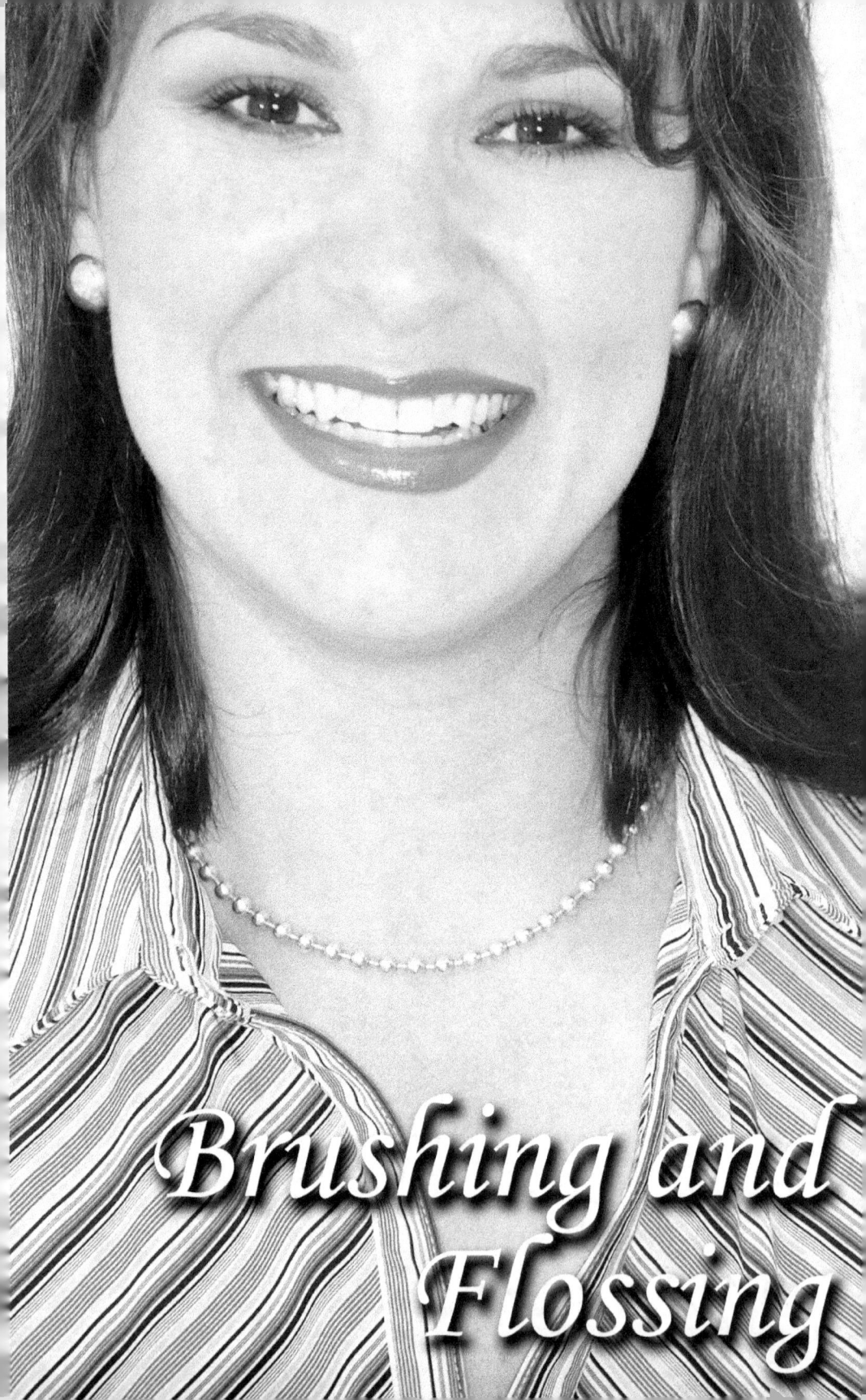

Brushing and Flossing

CHAPTER 11
Brushing and Flossing

Don't you love that just cleaned feeling of having teeth that are professionally cleaned? Your mouth feels as if it had an itch that's just been scratched. Your teeth feel smooth. Your breath feels fresh. It's a very pleasant feeling. Wouldn't you agree?

Well, you can't have a professional cleaning done everyday, right? Still, you need to keep your teeth and gums thoroughly cleaned up everyday. So what should you do on the home front on a regular basis?

I would be delighted if I could get my patients to do four things on a regular basis.

Number one, watch their diet. Don't eat things you know that are going to put you in danger, as far as your teeth or health is concerned.

Yes, it's fine to "cheat" occasionally, to enjoy yourself, but not to the point that it causes a detriment to your health or your teeth.

Sugary foods, juices, drinks, and other things that stick to your teeth with sugar in them put you in jeopardy. And a lot of people can't tolerate and get by with what they used to.

Remember, the more problems you've had in the past the closer you need to adhere to the principles of good home care and good diet.

Number two is to brush effectively. Sadly, the vast majority of the population, and I hope this doesn't include you, brushes somewhere between 20 and 50 seconds, with the average probably 30 seconds at a time.

They'll put a big ole wad of toothpaste on the end of their toothbrush, rub it around inside the mouth a few times and rinse it out. "Ah, my mouth feels better." That's really just a mouth wash.

My suggestion for using a toothbrush is, number one, always use one with soft bristles, not hard bristles.

While we used to think that hard bristles were better because they were stiffer and they "cleaned better." We now know it's just the opposite. You want the bristles of a toothbrush to clean below your gum. And the only way they can do that is to be soft enough that they will bend. As they bend, they reach down in that little space between the gum and the tooth where all the problems start for your gums.

A hard bristled brush or medium bristled brush simply won't bend enough to reach under where you need those bristles to go. So, you can't clean that area.

Number three is, angle your toothbrush at a 45 degree angle to the junction of your gum and your tooth. That's right, a 45 degree angle at the junction of your tooth and your gum. And when there, make little circles, little teeny, soft circles with your toothbrush systematically going through your mouth.

The double bonus is that this will clean the teeth and gums at the same time.

Number four: only use water or mouthwash to start each time you brush. I suggest to you that you brush twice. Once with water or mouthwash and then followed with a little toothpaste but no water. The first stage is only two minutes to mechanically clean off the invisible, sticky plaque. The second stage of a brushing can be your quickie in and out with toothpaste.

To brush, systematically start at one area of your mouth on the outside, come all the way around and then come back on the inside. Then do the same on the lower. Start on one side and work your way around all the way to the other side. And then come back on the

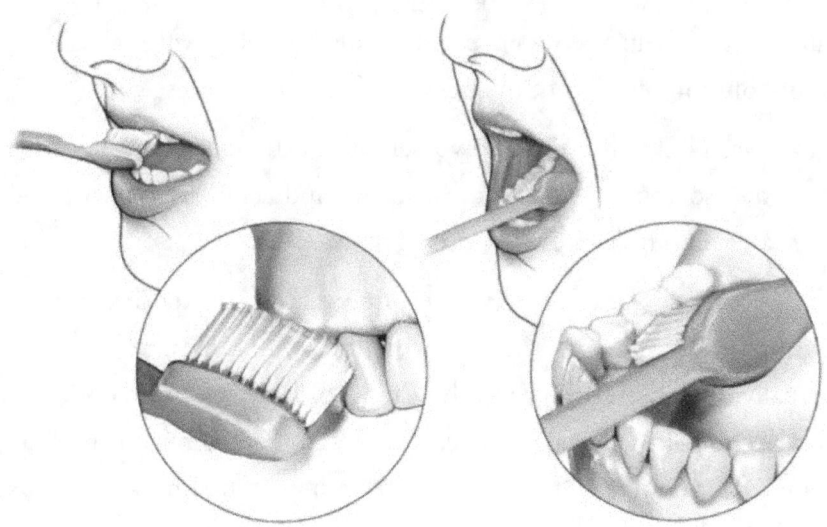

inside once again. This will complete a circuit that touches every tooth surface.

Don't worry about missing something on the tops of the teeth. In the process of cleaning the fronts and the backs of every tooth, that bristle will invariably get everything cleaned up on the tops too, like you need.

The next thing is understand what plaque is. What you're cleaning off is a sticky invisible substance. In fact, it's what is known as a biofilm. This biofilm resists all efforts to remove it. Your saliva has antibodies specifically designed to inhibit the bacteria that form plaque.

That's why those people with dry mouths, reduced salivary flow have more problems with gum disease and tooth decay, because the bacteria aren't inhibited by the saliva and the natural antibodies meant to fight them.

Many people have their mouths become dry as a result of aging, mouth-breathing and certain medications. In fact, there are well over 400 different medications that will dry your mouth when taking them.

If you have a dry mouth situation, you probably should get a saliva substitute to help keep your mouth moist. Sipping water all day is a good solution but it's not the best possible solution these days.

Warning: failing to keep your mouth extra clean and modifying your diet so you consume far less sugary and acidic things when you have a dry mouth can cause a dental disaster.

Plaque is the enemy. It's the thing that causes tooth decay and gum disease. And as I said, it's a biofilm, which means that plaque actually tries to hide underneath a "film" or layer that protects it from foods, moisture, antibodies, etc. That's why it requires mechanically removing the plaque from the teeth with physical implements like tooth brushing, floss, picks, etc. Irrigators do help but they aren't the final answer and do not substitute for mechanical removal. (I wish they did, too.)

So, to review, brush with water or mouth wash. Be systematic, go to every surface of the tooth, 45 degree angle to the tooth and the gum and make little circles.

I write "little circles" because I don't want you brushing back and forth. Brushing back and forth doesn't put the bristles in the place that they need to be. And it is more abrasive to the gum tissue.

By the way, I've had patients say to me, "I don't want to do it that way because I'm afraid it's going to make my gums recede." A point and fact: a soft brush, with a gentle touch, doesn't cause gum recession. Now if you brush like a banshee with a lot of force, anything will cause recession.

But the biggest reasons for recession, by the way, are one, dental plaque and two, aging.

Know this about plaque and why it's so destructive. It evolves. It changes in response to your efforts and your body's efforts to remove it.

It is a biofilm so it has a lot of protection. What we now know about biofilms is that these one celled bacteria ban together, and communicate with one another underneath that biofilm. They actually coordinate with each other to change shapes and change defenses to protect against attacks to remove them or kill them. It sounds pretty science fiction like, doesn't it?

Well, unfortunately that is the truth. The longer the plaque remains on the teeth the more destructive it becomes because the type of bacteria in the plaque, in that biofilm, evolves over time.

And that evolution from basically "good guy" bacteria to "very bad guy bacteria", the gum criminals, takes about 13 weeks. Which is why we tell most patients to come in about every 13 weeks. Every patient needs a customized schedule for maintenance care. These can range form two months to a year. For patients with a history of gum disease, every two to three months is about right. If you have had no history of gum disease, those intervals are every 4 to 6 months. And then rarely, a teeny percentage can come yearly.

For most people I suggest using a power tooth brush. A power brush has a two minute timer on it. It has thousands of strokes per minute and it has the right consistency of bristle. It's not too hard, not too soft. For many, that increased efficiency of cleaning one's own mouth by using a power brush can mean the difference between good check-ups and bad ones.

Flossing

Flossing: dentists always talk about it, patients seem to hate it.

"I can't figure out how to use it." "It's not convenient for me to use it." "It seems like it's too hard."

Well, I suggest to you that you get an education from your dentist about how to floss again, if you're still having trouble. There are certain floss holders that can be helpful. But I would encourage you to learn about what we call magic flossing fingers. That literally means wrapping the floss, about 18 inches of it, around your middle fingers and then systematically using your index finger and thumb to maneuver among the teeth. Have your dentist or hygienist demonstrate how to use it so it doesn't frustrate you or feel you must lie to your dentist about how often you use it! Once you know how and practice a little, it becomes very easy and quite fast.

Now, for me, I'm not wedded to the idea that you must floss. I know that sounds like dental blasphemy, but here's the reality. Over 9 in 10 Americans do not floss regularly or consistently. One figure I heard was 92%.

So, if you're not going to floss, what should you use?

Well, you can use a product called a Stimudent or a Proxabrush. Use something to get in between your teeth. Why?

Because 85% of all problems for adults occur between the teeth. That's where floss cleans. Only 15% of the problems occur on the biting surface or on the smooth surfaces of the teeth where you normally brush. Wow, that means flossing is more important than my brushing? Well, the answer is yes. You should actually start your home care by flossing your teeth first, followed by brushing.

When you don't clean between your teeth, the plaque evolves and gets more destructive to your gums and teeth. It causes an inflammatory response from the infection that courses through your body, worsening a multitude of conditions and diseases.

After it has remained on the teeth and roots for a while, it starts to calcify creating what most people call dental tartar. We call it calculus.

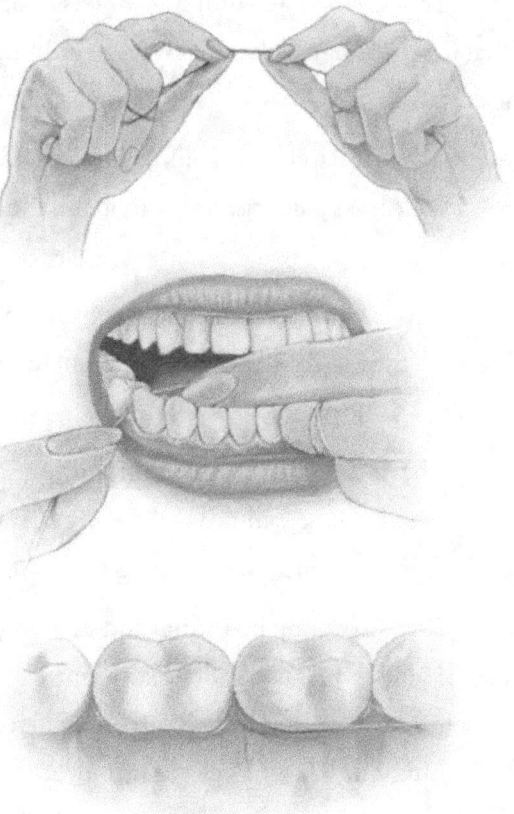

Dental tartar tends to accumulate where saliva comes out of the ducts in your mouth. There are six places where that occurs. And it's those six places where the most calculus or tartar develops.

The calculus is particularly challenging for you to clean and for your body to tolerate. Plaque accumulates on calculus and it's very difficult to get off. The calculus acts like a foreign body meaning it doesn't belong. So, it's important for that tartar or calculus to come off. If you have built up calculus, you body will love having it removed so it has a chance to start healing.

Failure to See A Need

One of the reasons that people don't come and see a dentist on a regular basis is because they fail to see a need. Many may say, "I'm not in any pain. Why do I need to see a dentist?"

Boy, is that bad thinking. It gets people in trouble. And the more that this thought pervades your thinking, the more trouble you're going to have.

Unfortunately, you don't have the same capacity to keep your mouth clean as a dentist and a hygienist . So they are necessary for your dental health.

If your gums bleed when you brush or floss, it doesn't mean to stop. It means that the gums are so inflamed that they bleed when brushed or flossed.

The more you floss correctly, the more you brush correctly, the less bleeding you will have. It will generally only take a few days of cleaning well before the bleeding stops.

If, in spite of brushing and flossing correctly, your gums still bleed, you should see a dentist. Come and see us right away, because you may have other problems or incorrect techniques or something else going on. We will help you find out what that is. Delaying can be costly in terms of comfort, health and what it costs to get corrected.

Seeing your dentist on a regular basis and receiving maintenance care helps you to not only keep your teeth, but your overall health is preserved. And that's what it's all about, isn't it? With what we know now about the connections between your oral conditions and the rest of your body, it is a deadly gamble to put off or delay needed dental care.

Amanda's Story

When Amanda first showed up in my office, I knew she had something special about her. Maybe it was the way that she spoke or carried herself, but I knew there was something special about her. Amanda had grown up overseas. She was the daughter of missionary parents. Her parents had been missionaries in Africa and Asia, and she had finally come to the states to go to college. As you might imagine, coming from missionary parents, they didn't have a whole lot of money. And as you also might imagine, the dentistry she'd had growing up wasn't all that good in those third world countries.

So here she was in front of me now, telling me about what she wanted for her mouth. I couldn't quite figure out why I couldn't see her teeth. Amanda had gotten through school by working her way through, and had just taken a new job, a good job.

Then she showed me what was going on. The reason we couldn't see her teeth was because they were decayed and broken. She was a "train wreck", that's what she called it.

She said, "Look. I'll do anything I need to do to get my teeth back looking like they need to. 'Cause I know how important it is to my life and my health. You figure out what needs to be done and I'll figure out what needs to be done so I can get it paid for. Will you help me?"

Well, our heart went out to her, because we knew this was a person who needed what we can do and needed it badly. After quite a bit of working it out and months of care, Amanda had her smile back.

She could chew again, so she went off the fattening, soft foods. She'd lost 20 pounds and now she carried herself even better. She looked like she could run for the senate.

I said, "Amanda, you've paid us. You've been a great patient and we know you've made some sacrifices to get it done. What did you do? How did you manage to get to do this?"

And then she related that she had taken a second job, borrowed the money so she could get the work done. She didn't have the advantage that many people have of being able to go and get money from the credit union or getting a home equity loan. She didn't have stocks she could sell or CDs stocked away in the bank. She went and got another job.

I said, "Amanda, how are you doing now?"

She said, "Great. I've gotten two promotions in my original job and I'm about to move."

I said, "Where are you going?"

"New York"

I said, "Well, good luck."

She smiled, "Well, a lot of it is because of what you guys did for me. So, thank you so much."

Amanda is now working for a major advertising firm in New York City and doing fabulously well. Privacy rules prevent me from telling you all there is to know. Let's just say you've seen her work if you've watched any television.

Portrait Photography and Dentistry
by Dr. Joe Marcius

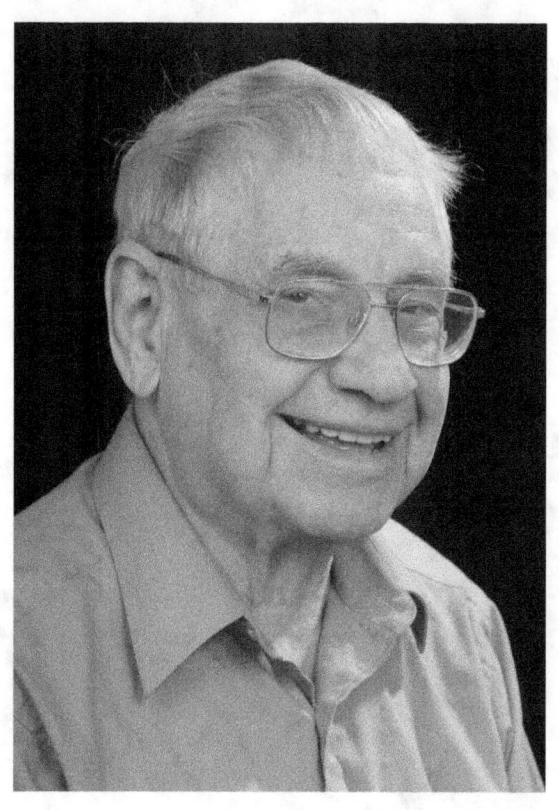

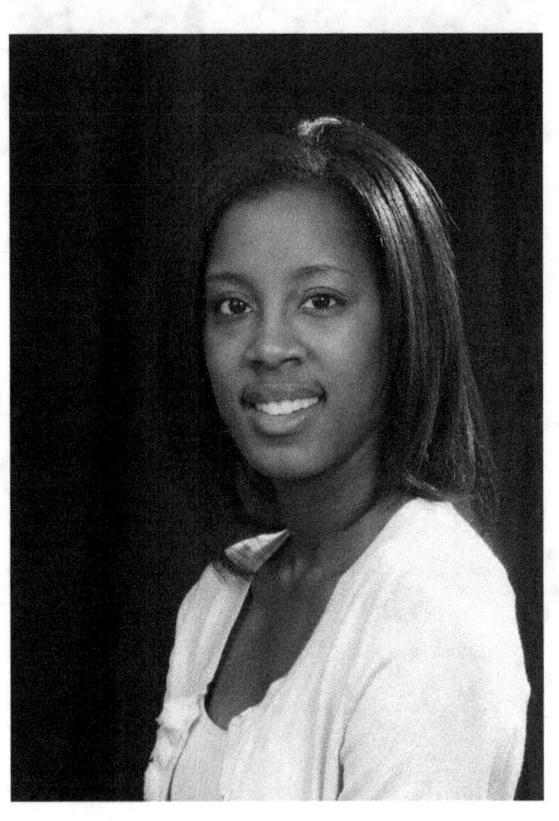

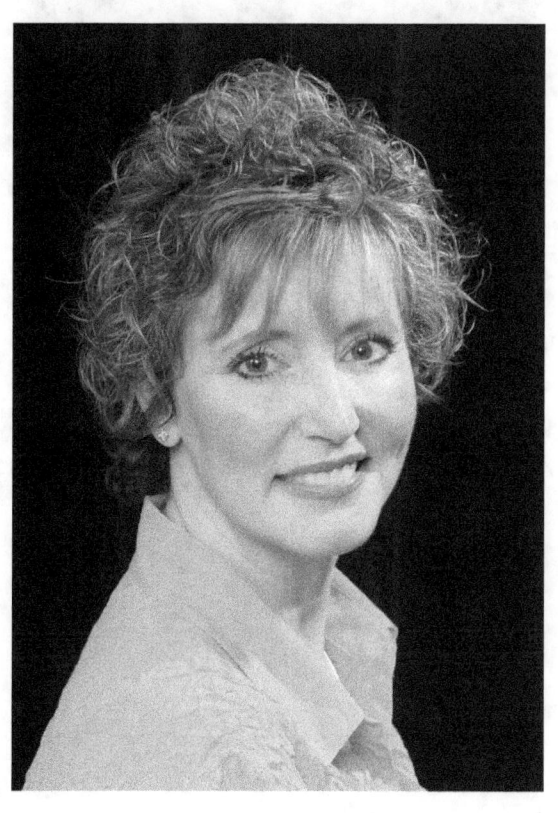

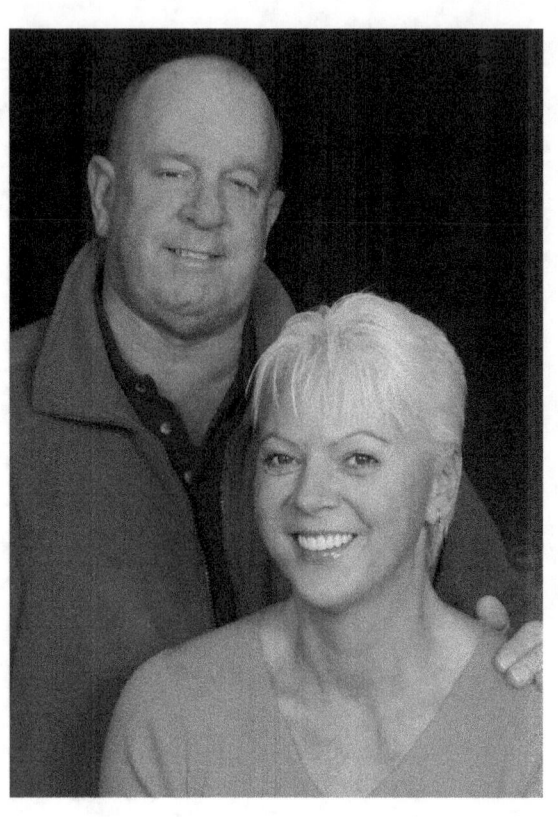

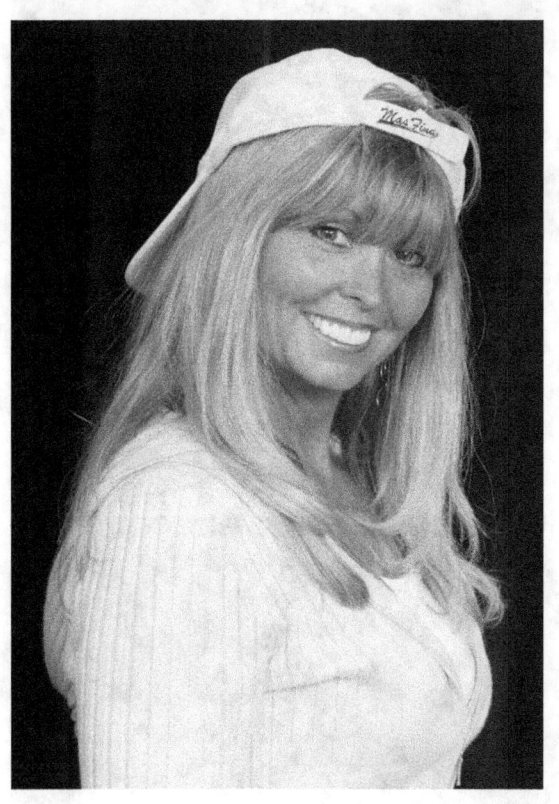

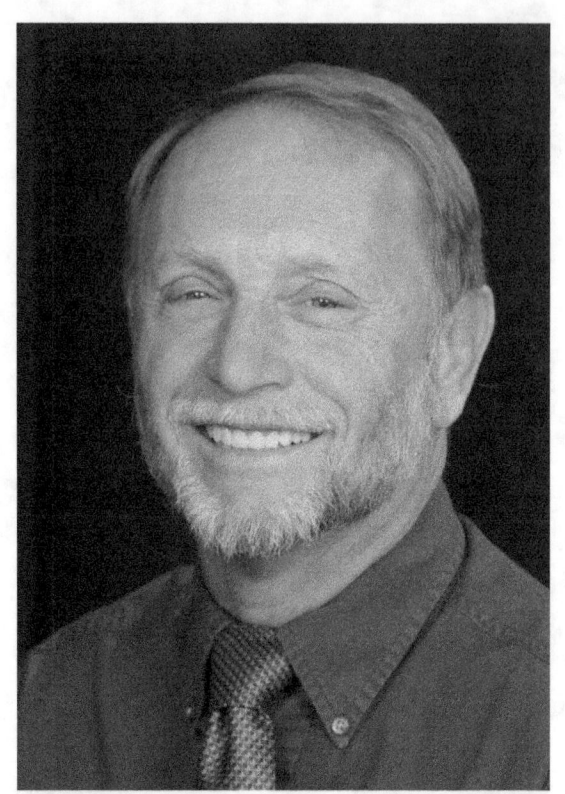

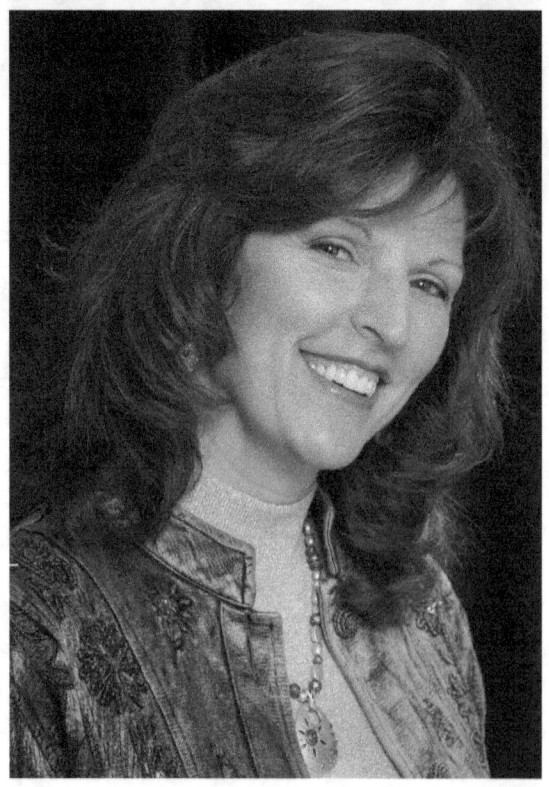

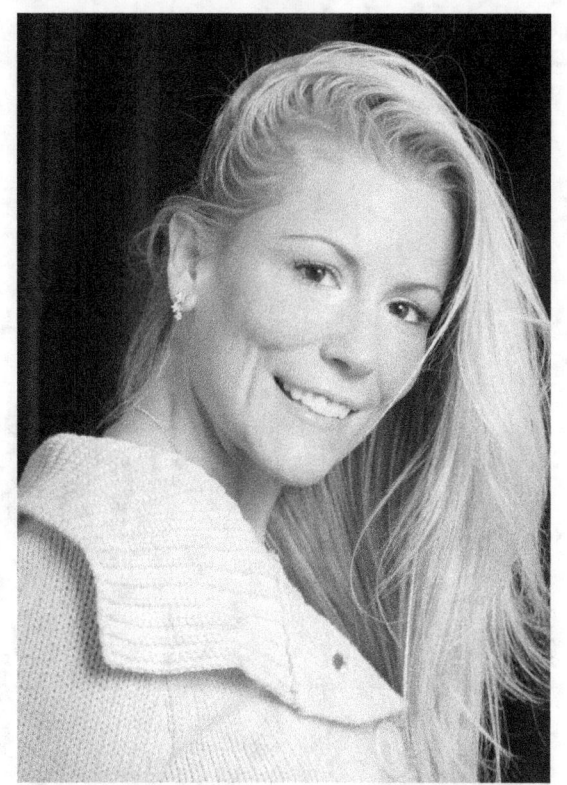

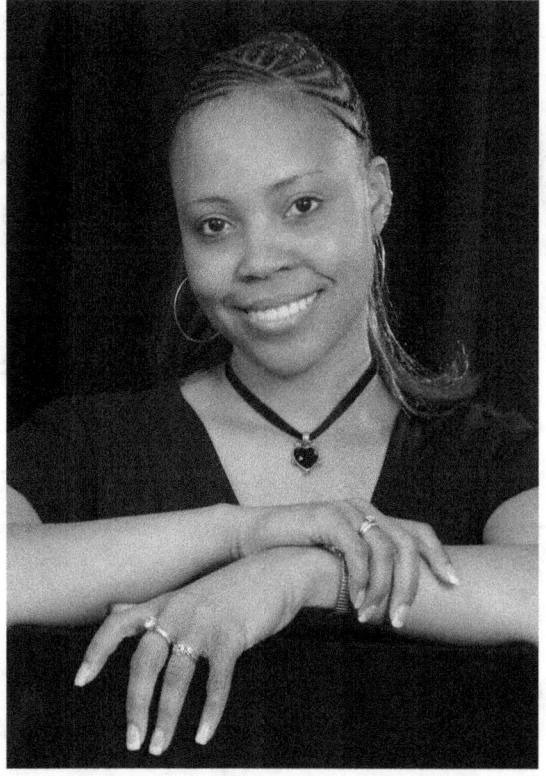

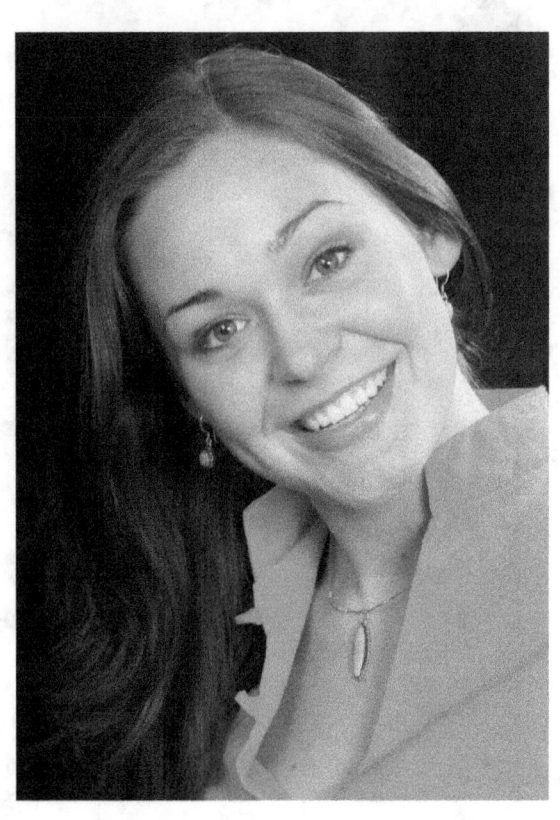

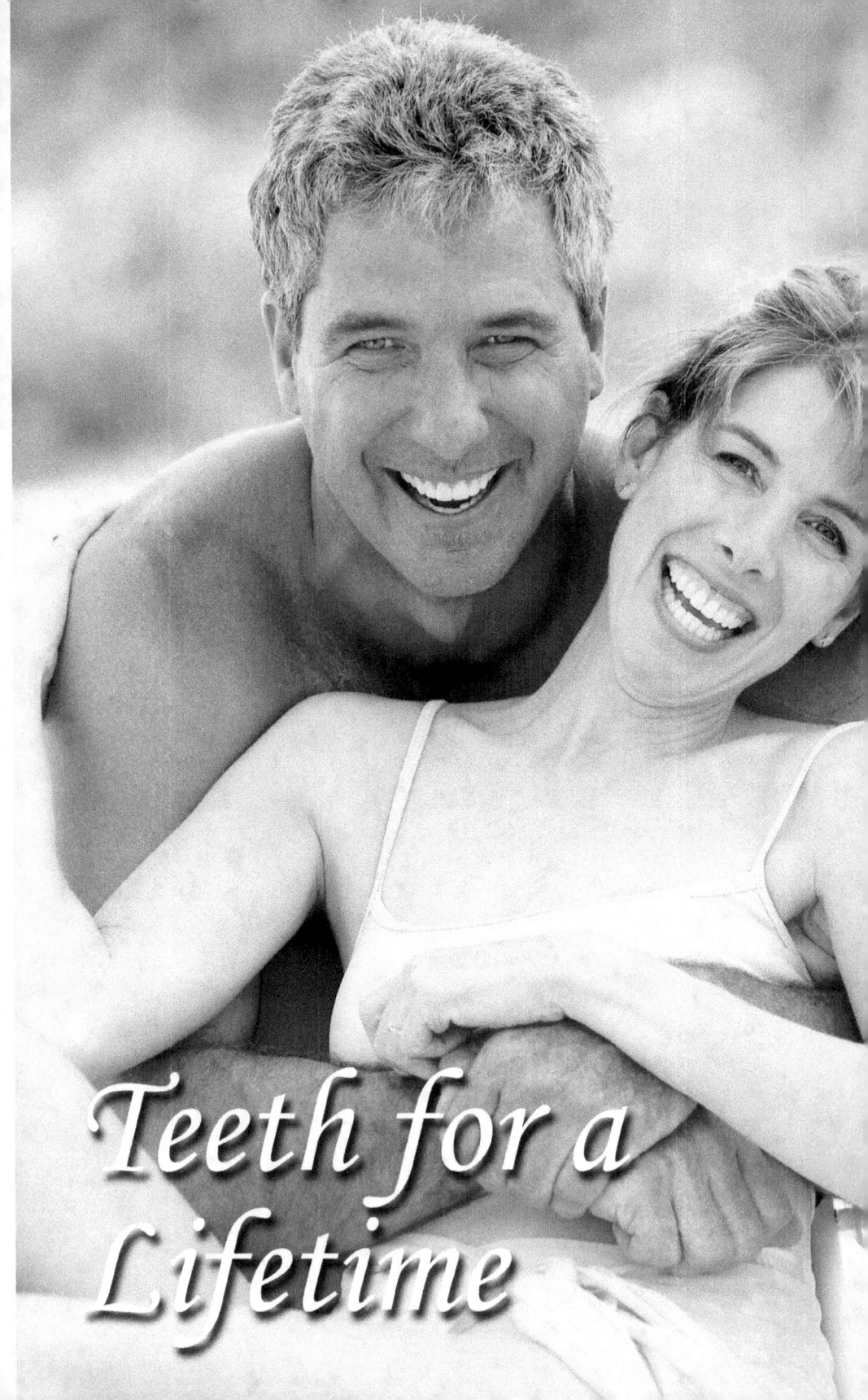

Teeth for a Lifetime

CHAPTER 12
How to Keep Your Teeth for a Lifetime
Helping Babies and Small Children

Let's start at the beginning. From birth to two years of age is a time of multiple physicians' visits, of great joy, of sleepy moms and dads and a whole lot of learning about life while being tired.

If you're a parent or grandparent, you know what I'm talking about.

During this time the baby has a natural sucking instinct. That's a good thing. That's how he learns to eat. For many moms who are nursing, once the teeth erupt into the mouth, nursing stops.

We dentists are suggesting that you begin to get the baby accustomed to cleaning the mouth early on. Obviously, in the first few months, there are no teeth in the mouth to clean. It's important to use a clean damp cloth to wipe off the gums at this stage to get the baby accustomed to having someone in his mouth keeping it clean.

Expect your children to get their first teeth around five to nine months. The first will be the front teeth, usually the lower front teeth.

Use a clean, warm, damp washcloth and wipe the gums clean until the teeth come in. Then, as soon as the teeth start coming in, you should start using a baby sized toothbrush with soft bristles to brush the teeth.

You as the parent or grandparent should brush the baby's teeth. You are instilling a good habit.

Begin bringing the toddler into the dentist at around age 18 months. Think of it as an orientation. The toddler gets accustomed to the sights, sounds and smells, and gets on the right road to creating trust with the dentist. It's also a good opportunity to review the child's diet.

We want every small child to start off with a positive dental experience.

When you wait until three or four years old to bring a child to a dentist, particularly when there's a problem, it makes it very difficult for a small child to rationally think about the situation. And he can equate going to the dentist with things like going to the pediatrician to have a shot. Not something they like.

It's also important, as a parent or a grandparent, to understand that your dental health has a direct effect on the baby because you'll very likely to share cups and spoons and glasses and all kinds of things with that child. Through these shared foods and drinks, you can transmit the bacteria that causes gum disease and tooth decay to that child!

So, it's important for you, mom and dad, grand moms and grand dads, to make sure that your mouths are in good shape.

One of the most important things you do for an infant, at this early age, is to prevent them from going to bed with a bottle that has soda, juice, milk or even formula, because it could subject the child to what I call 'baby bottle decay.'

Baby bottle decay is ugly, and traumatic. It can cause serious problems and often requires a hospital visit to first remove decay and subsequently cover the stumps with strange looking silver colored teeth on top of the small child's teeth. This isn't something we like to do, but it is better than the child suffering from all that decay.

If you're going to put a child to bed with a bottle, make sure that you do so with water in the bottle. That will not cause decay.

Understand that when babies teethe they can be grumpy. They will be more irritable. They can be restless, have a loss of appetite and cry.

It can help, during this time when they're teething, to use that clean damp cloth and gently massage the gums. This can help relieve some of the teething discomfort. You can also try using a chilled teething toy or some teething gel. This will have the dual benefit of comforting the child and speeding the eruption of the primary (baby) teeth.

Here's a sure road to failure - telling the child not to be afraid. Children can't differentiate the word "not" very well. And they'll likely only hear the word, "afraid."

After that first visit, you should bring your child to see the dentist about every six months for professional cleanings and exams.

From approximately age two to seven, many kids receive preventative care, sealants for the first molars, repairs to the teeth, even observation for possible orthodontic treatment.

It's important that parents continue to help small children with brushing after meals, and put a heavy emphasis on avoiding foods with sugar, or ones that stick to the teeth.

The rest of the primary, or baby teeth, usually erupt by age six. For some, it happens as early as age five. There will be ten teeth on the top, ten on the bottom.

If there are spaces between the primary teeth, there's no need to worry because the spacing helps create room for the permanent teeth that are coming in behind them. The baby teeth provide the ability for a small child to eat normally, be considered sociably acceptable among other small children and provide the matrix, if you will, for the growth of the permanent teeth.

If there is crowding in baby teeth at a young age, there will probably be crowding in the permanent teeth later on. Understand, by the way, that sucking on a finger or thumb up until about age three is considered within normal range. Beyond that time can change the growth pattern and development of the teeth and jaws. You should actively work with your child and your dentist to stop it as soon as possible after age three.

The important thing for a small child is getting off on a good start. This includes eating the right foods and avoiding sugary drinks, especially soft drinks, sugared waters and some juices.

Be careful with fluoride supplements and even fluoridated water. Some formulas have fluoride built into them. So make sure that the fluoride content of your water doesn't mix with the fluoride content that could be in a formula. Excessive fluoride can cause fluorosis, which causes white spots on teeth and can cause teeth to be more prone to decay. If you live in a community with fluoridated water, you probably won't need the fluoride supplementation for your child.

One common dental problem for a small child is called thrush: a fungal infection that results in a tender, red, inflamed mouth. It can even affect their mother. During breastfeeding a mother can re-infect the child and the child can even re-infect the mom, resulting in itching and redness of the breasts, and even burning and shooting pains in the breasts. Your dentist or physician can help you manage this if it happens to your child.

Another thing that occasionally occurs is called Epstein's pearls. These arrive early in the life of an infant. Epstein's Pearls are hardened pads that occur on the gums and palate. This tissue helps the baby latch onto mom's breast while nursing. They could be called 'suckling pads.' The problem occurs when these pads become swollen and hard.

Though they may be uncomfortable, there's really nothing to worry about because these will shed in time.

Once all of a child's teeth come in, it's important to monitor them. Come to the dentist every six months to get their teeth professionally cleaned, and if possible, floss your children's teeth for them.

Follow these toothbrush tips: Don't share your toothbrush with your kids, and replace theirs every two to four months. If your child has a cold or flu, make sure that you get the child a new toothbrush. Throw the old one away. And store all toothbrushes so they don't touch each other, not in a glass where they all mingle.

If for some reason a baby has an accident of some sort and knocks a baby tooth out, do not try to reinsert it back into the mouth. Instead, call the dentist immediately.

Between ages six and twelve, while many primary teeth remain, the lower, permanent, first molars arrive. These are the keystones to the development of the upper and lower jaw. So, they're important to keep healthy.

Dentists call this period 'mixed dentition,' which literally means the mouth has primary teeth and permanent teeth simultaneously.

Fortunately, some of the primary teeth are larger than the permanent teeth and actually create room for the permanent teeth as the jaws grow.

Most children will still benefit greatly from having orthodontic treatment. And somewhere around age seven is when most should have an orthodontic evaluation.

Often, the shape of the jaws can be altered at this time with different types of orthodontics to help create space for teeth that will come.

This period is also the time to set good habits. Make sure that the child is brushing at least a couple of times a day and flossing at least once. Usually the parent will help with the flossing.

By age twelve most children's adult teeth are in place. If orthodontics are planned, this is a good time to do it. Typically, between age 12 and 17, orthodontics should be completed. Often girls are ready before boys due to growth and eruption patterns being earlier in girls.

This general period, from age 7 to 18, is also a good time to apply sealants. Sealants are special plastics that seal the grooves in the back teeth off so bacteria can't get down into the grooves and cause decay.

It's also the time when wisdom teeth often erupt. Often these teeth need to be removed for purposes of maintaining tooth position and prevent future problems. Teenagers typically recover from third molar surgery pretty fast. The longer they wait, the more difficult it becomes.

This is also the time when a child's first cold sores can develop. These are triggered by fevers or physical and emotional stresses, even excessive exposure to the sun. These cold sores are typically viral in nature. If they get bad enough, your dentist can prescribe certain antiviral treatments.

A particular concern during this time is teenage bulimia. Bulimia is an eating disorder where the afflicted deliberately vomits to keep weight down. As you might imagine, stomach acid can be quite toxic to the teeth and can lead to severe erosion of the teeth. Your dentist can diagnose this and in some cases may be the first to spot the condition. Active intervention is a must because bulimia can become life threatening.

For the most part, as a parent or grandparent, just be watchful of your teenager and their dental health. Make sure that they are being diligent with their home care and diet.

Create a safe food environment for them. Don't stock the refrigerator with sodas and ice cream or candies and sweets. If you do, you're just asking for it.

And if your children are involved in athletics, encourage them to use protective mouth guards. I have seen more mouth injuries from children playing soccer and baseball than youth league football. I believe the reason is that the young football players are forced to wear protective athletic mouthguards, while the other kids are not. I suggest that every child involved in contact sports, including contact from a ball coming in at high speeds, should wear a protective athletic mouthguard.

Age 18-32: The Danger Years

Years 18 to 32 are what I call the danger years. Teenagers grow up to become adults. They go off to college and get jobs. They meet the love of their life and move around a lot. So, there are a lot more exciting things happening than their oral health.

It's a period where many people avoid the dentist because there's nobody there reminding them or making appointments for them. They may think they don't have the money for the dentist. So, not surprisingly, this is a time when dental health can decline significantly.

You, as a parent or grandparent, can help stop this with reminders, both gentle and not so gentle. Make sure these young adults see the dentist so all the work you did to preserve their teeth early on doesn't go to waste. Preventive maintenance can go a very long way for the young adults of this age.

Age 32-40: The Return to Regular Dental Care

On the other hand, a large percentage of adults start going back to the dentist on a regular basis from ages 32 to 40. Some feel a little guilty for having ignored their teeth. As you can imagine, people of this age group often need to have a lot of repair work performed so problems don't get worse.

It's interesting, we often see adults about this age using their children as scouts to check out a dentist before they come in themselves for their own care.

Age 32 to 40 is also a time when some teeth have gotten so bad they must be removed. And the time when an unfortunate few just give up on their teeth and have dentures placed. Whatever you do, don't make this mistake unless your teeth are terminal and keeping them threatens your jaw health and health as a whole.

On the brighter side, it's at this age that minor corrections such as tooth whitening or cosmetic bonding can help change a tooth's look and make a big difference in your appearance.

Here's something to understand in the chronology of life and your dentistry: The dental sins of the past do accumulate. What you can tolerate physically when you were younger, you often can't as you age. And the absence of pain doesn't mean there aren't problems. In fact, pain is usually a late indicator of trouble. While pain does indicate a problem, the absence of pain does not indicate everything is okay. If you have no pain, you can still have problems.

Also, understand that when you lose a tooth, it is not a single tooth event. Multiple teeth move to compensate for the loss of that one tooth. This compensation throws off the bite mechanism and amplifies the possibility of gum disease, the loss of more teeth and makes a mismatch in the bite. Moreover, the teeth that have moved are more likely to get cavities because they trap food and are harder to keep clean.

And appreciate that your gums bleeding when you brush IS a big deal. If you don't clean between your teeth, you will have problems because there – beyond the reach of the toothbrush – is where the vast majority of adult dental problems occur.

Throwing in the towel on your teeth is always a bad move if you can prevent it. We see many, many people who come to us after they have given up on their teeth. Gratefully, we can usually help them reclaim teeth that look good and feel good again.

Age 40 and Beyond: Aging Teeth

By the time someone's 40, they usually encounter more significant problems that they can see and feel due to problems accumulated from the past: incomplete care, patchwork dentistry, or work never done in the first place.

Because problems with your teeth accumulate over time you can have significant gum disease and breakdown of old restorations as you grow older. Fillings fall apart. And while typically your concern shifts to your children and ensuring they get orthodontics and the complete care that they need, you often neglect yourself.

Yet, for you to be the best mom or dad you need to be, you should make sure that your teeth are in good health. 40 is about the age that the 200% to 400% rule kicks in: for every year you needed care but didn't get it, you'll spend two to four times the typical annual limit of your dental insurance.

As I write this, that annual limit typically amounts to $1,500 a year. If you do the math, that means it could take $3,000 to $6,000 for every year needed treatment is neglected.

 For more information go to: http://www.pubmedcentral.nih.gov/articlerender.fcgi?article=1448334

That's ugly news. But it's reality. And hopefully, the kick you need to get the care you need. While prevention creates relatively small financial issues, major corrections can create big financial issues. Ignoring things threatens your dental health, and greatly threatens your overall health.

Around age 40 to 45 is when a lot of marriages begin to come apart and smiles actually become more important. It's something we notice at my office. Forty-something divorcees are often prime candidates for cosmetic dentistry and smile makeovers. And frankly, we do a lot of them.

By 50, the accumulated neglect and patchwork dentistry takes its toll . The teeth are even worse. Stains on the teeth become common and "set in", teeth drift to new positions, and people experience chronic bad breath and gum disease. And while poor eating habits cause some new decay, many people of this age take medications that cause them to have less salivary flow. In other words, their mouth is dry. They have no saliva to help protect their teeth.

This is also the time when you can get a very large payback in doing something about the situation. You could have much longer to live. For many, having healthy teeth will mean an entirely different life in their later years; more zestful living, a better diet and better health. For some it could mean staying out of nursing homes.

So, even if you have a mouth full of problems, you can solve them. And giving up is not a good strategy. Nor is hoping things will get better by themselves.

If you are 60+, you should assess the health of your teeth. You are going to need them for a long time. Over half those age 60 will live to be in their 90's or older.

The thought of having to live your life with permanent mouth disabilities should give you pause. For some, this age can mean a revitalization and rejuvenation of overall health.

More than once have we helped someone in their 70's and even 80's to get their teeth rebuilt, and as a result, avoid chronic health problems.

Also, one out of five folks over age 60 is diabetic. This number is only expected to climb. Type 2 diabetes makes your dental health worse and poor dental health worsens one's ability to control the diabetes. Moreover, there are over 57 million pre-diabetics.

To really stay ahead of all of these possible hurdles, it's important to get your teeth in good health, so you can live your best life.

Isn't that what it's all about?

Dreama's Story

I want to tell the story about the patient who said no and then came back years later.

We'd first seen Dreama when she was 38 years old. We could say she'd had a hard time in life. She grew up in a lower middle class family with not a whole lot, with infrequent visits to the dentist, and had a huge sweet tooth. When we first saw her, she had a mouth full of cavities and her smile was suffering because of it. And so was her self esteem. We told Dreama everything that she needed to do, and she decided not to see us. She chose to do something else.

When she walked back into our office, seven years later it was far worse. She had opted to find the cheapest route possible. She had lost a lot of teeth and had patchwork dentistry done. Patchwork dentistry is sort of like scotch taping teeth back together. It helps out a little while, but it doesn't last all that long.

Dreama was now back in our office and saying, "I'm so sorry I didn't choose to work with you. Huge mistake on my part. Will you take me back?"

Well, not only did we take Dreama back; we helped her recover from her mistakes of the past and put her back together again. She got the great smile she always wanted.

Dreama is now 46 years old, recently married to the man that she always wanted to marry. She now smiles brightly and tells us about the trips she takes. We wish we could do all those trips.

When Dreama came back to us, she confided that when she originally came to us years earlier that she'd talked to a friend about what she was about to do and how much it would cost. Her well-meaning friend had said she'd be crazy to spend that money on her teeth to get them fixed.

Dreama lived to regret listening to her friend.

 She finally got it fixed, but first suffered all that anguish, pain and added expense because of trying to go cheap. Her friend was well meaning, but didn't know the depths of Dreama's problems. Her friend advised from her own experience. Dreama's were so much more severe. Unfortunately, this is all too common.

Dreama didn't know then what she knows now.

She told us this, "Please tell my story so other people don't make the mistake I made."

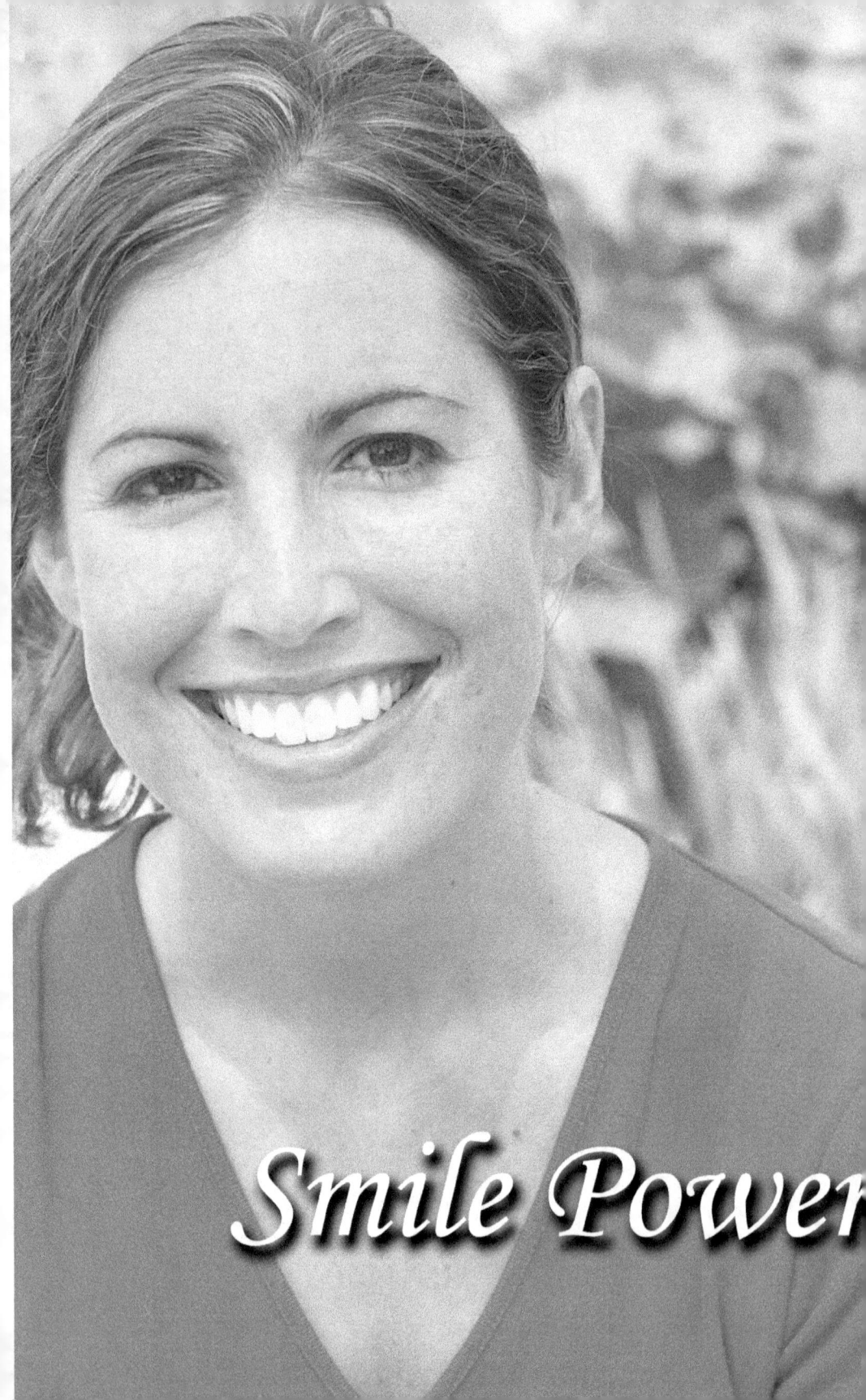

Smile Power

CHAPTER 13
Smile Power
Cosmetic Dentistry To The Rescue

Are you proud of your smile? When was the last time you smiled ear to ear for a camera? Do you receive compliments on your smile? Can your smile light up a room just by walking into it?

If you said "No" to any one of these questions, you may want to consider changing your smile fortune. Fortune is a particularly good word here.

Why? Because your smile can be worth a fortune to you over your lifetime. What kind of fortune? A beauty fortune , a health fortune, a financial fortune, a relationship fortune and a fortune in how you feel about yourself.

Being smile wealthy is a particularly joyous condition because your smile is with you 24/7 365 days a year for your lifetime. Sounds like a pretty good investment, doesn't it?

So, your smile can be either a fortune or a misfortune that haunts you, causing you to always wish for a different one, a better one, one that you can beam at everyone you meet.

Wouldn't it be better to be proud of your smile, knowing that you look great whenever you use it? Can you imagine the difference it could make for you?

You might know someone who is seemingly unaffected by his or her smile, even though it doesn't look so great. Some people just don't seem to be bothered by their smile. If you or someone you know doesn't have a good looking smile and feels okay with it, you may not want to do anything about being smile-challenged. Then again, once you know more, you might want to reconsider.

You may already know that your smile is "challenged." You may even realize that it's a handicap, a disability of sorts. It need not be this way.

Why live with this disability when it can be fixed? Why live with it when you can turn that disability actually into an asset?

Cosmetic dentistry today is different than it used to be. With the technology, science, understanding and art, you aren't stuck any more like you used to be. I can still remember patients coming to me years ago saying, "I don't want that black line up around my gums when I have a crown placed in the front." That was long ago.

At one point in time dentistry didn't have a solution for that problem. Now we do.

You can actually get teeth that look like teeth – beautiful, white teeth that give you a great smile.

Lessons from History

What you may not know is that having a good-looking smile has been important for thousands of years. From Egyptian Pharaohs, to the Inca Indians, appearance was important.

The Pharaohs would often attempt to borrow a tooth from a slave to place in their own mouth after they had lost one. These failed because the teeth were rejected.

The Incas were famous for placing inlays of precious jewels into their teeth. That was considered attractive and a sign of importance.

Today, as we learn more and more about your teeth, your smile and its relationship to your health and your whole body, cosmetic dentistry is more than just about looking good.

Back then, you didn't need your teeth as long. The average lifespan at the time of Alexander the Great was just 21 years old! That's why older people were admired and respected so much. People figured anyone who could figure out how to live a long time must have something special about them.

At the time that the social security system was developed in the 20th century, the average lifespan was 47 years. Now we're hitting 80+ and it's rising quickly.

So, teeth used to matter less. They matter more now because you are going to be around longer and you're going to need your teeth longer.

Luckily, we have the ability to do something about the appearance and utility of older teeth.

Here are some things you should know. Your teeth darken naturally as you grow older. This comes as a result of the foods that we eat and things that we drink that stain your teeth.

We can now reverse that process.

Here's something that people don't realize. Pretty teeth are functional teeth, too. When teeth are in the right position, they naturally deflect food away from the gums. Teeth that are correctly positioned help you keep your mouth cleaner and makes them easier to take care of.

When the teeth are in a correct bite position, the smile looks better. When they're in correct alignment, they not only look better, but they distribute the force of chewing along all the teeth – which literally reduces stress to your teeth.

I think celebrities know things about their smiles that most people don't. They understand that how their smile looks is critical to their success.

What you may not know is your own appearance is critical to your success.

Having the right smile for you is more important now than ever. Your smile should match your personality, the proportions of your face, the shape of your face, and even the height of your body.

We know that your smile power has a direct effect on how other people perceive you, and how you perceive yourself. It even affects how teachers respond to small children in school.

A study found that children who looked better were treated more favorably by teachers.

Even prisoners who looked better in a court room received more favorable sentences than those who did not.

Some of the effects of looking good:

- Attracting the romantic partner of your dreams.

- Looking up to 10 years younger.

- Ability to eat what your heart desires including steak, corn-on-the-cob, apples, caramel, and more.

- The more beautiful your smile, the less people notice thin lips, a receding hairline, a too-large nose, pimples or gray hair.

- Developing more self-confidence.

- Keeping your teeth for a lifetime.

- Having fewer illnesses.

Your smile is something that's with you 24/7. How often you use that smile is part of your communication. You use it to make others feel comfortable with you and to influence. It determines a great deal for you on a whole number of levels.

For some it can mean a rekindling of romance. It can mean a relationship blossomed that would have never had a chance before.

It can be a personal rejuvenation in how you feel about yourself. And with that, how others feel about you, too.

Your beaming smile can help you get the promotion by looking the part. And for many, it helps to keep that 'edge.' It's about beating the competition.

Your smile helps to create a youthful look.

It may be the ultimate anti-aging tool, which brings me to this point: What do people look at when they look at your face? We used to think it was kind of a 50/50 trade off. That 50% of the time people are looking at your eyes and 50% of the time they're looking at your smile.

We now know, from more recent studies, that **81% of people consider the smile to be the most important part of facial appearance**.

Startling isn't it?

What happens when you hide your smile? How do you feel about you? And how do others feel about you?

Think about that. When you meet new people and if you're hiding your smile, they may look at you and say to themselves, "What's wrong with you?" Or "What's wrong with me?" Either way that relationship or friendship is inhibited – sometimes fatally. Who knows how many budding relationships are killed by an hidden smile?

Are you a candidate for cosmetic dentistry?

- Are you confident about your smile?
- Are you comfortable in smiling broadly around other people?
- Do you keep your mouth closed when you feel it might reveal your smile?
- Do you wish you had a smile as nice as someone you know at work or in social settings?
- Do you ever use your hand to hide your smile?
- Do you ever find yourself drawn to pictures of people with beautiful smiles?
- Have you ever felt you wanted a smile like a fashion model or a celebrity?
- Do you feel your smile makes you look older than you actually are?
- When you look at your smile in the mirror, are you proud of what you see?
- Does your present smile make you look confident or less confident?
- Do you notice other people's smiles when you meet them?
- Do you find yourself looking at your smile and wishing it looked better?
- Do you want your teeth to be whiter?
- Are you happy with the appearance of your gums?
- Do you find yourself saying, "I want a pretty smile" or "I wish I had a better smile?"
- Do you show too much or too little teeth when you smile?
- Does some small imperfection in your smile bother you?
- Do you sometimes wish for gums that showed less or showed more when you smile?
- Do you show enough teeth when you smile?
- Would you want teeth that are longer or shorter, narrower or wider, more rounded or more square?
- Does your smile fit your personality?
- Would you want a smile that makes you look 10 to 15 years younger than you actually are?
- Carefully review your answers because they will be telling.

What Celebrities Know

Celebrities have cosmetic dentistry done because they also know it can literally transform their careers. There are quite a few very well known actors whose career took off after they had their smile transformations.

People who won't fix other parts of their appearance fix their teeth.

Donald Trump doesn't fix his hair. He can certainly afford it. But check out his teeth. His smile looks good, even if he doesn't show it very often. His hair has become a sort of trademark. He knew better with his smile. He now looks like a different person when he is smiling.

Vanity or the New Necessity?

Of course, some consider it a bit vain to be concerned about their appearance. It really isn't at all. We know better now. We know how your smile affects other people. We know how it affects your influence. We know how it affects how other people treat you.

And what's possible now is that virtually everyone could have a good looking smile.

The new rule is: if you can imagine it, it's probably possible.

Whether you need a smile enhancement or a complete smile makeover, cosmetic dentistry now has the tools and technology to bring you the smile you've always wanted. Of course, that's assuming you're seeing a dentist who's trained, and has the experience, training and talent for performing cosmetic dentistry.

Let me tell you about Harold. When he came to me, he was 28 years old, had graduated from college, and had entered a managerial training program. He had done pretty well for himself. But he had become a bit disgruntled with his job prospects with that particular company and decided to quit.

When he came to me he wanted to look better. Now frankly, Harold's problems were pretty small. He didn't need a lot of work to make him look better.

For Harold the work was whitening his teeth and doing some cosmetic contouring of individual front teeth to create the proper contours and shapes.

The result: a happier, more confident Harold. The second result: he went out and found the job that he had really wanted when he first graduated college.

And now he happily returns to us for his regular maintenance and smiles all the time. A happy ending. An appropriate treatment for an appropriate situation.

Jean, on the other hand, was a mess when she came to see us. She knew she was a mess. And she did not want to look that way anymore.

She was in her late 30's, still unmarried and unfortunately, her teeth had taken a turn for the worse. They were dark and she'd had a lot of old fillings that just plain didn't look good.

Jean was far from just being smile challenged, she had a true smile handicap.

She told me that she often put her hand in front of her face instead of smiling proudly. After that she withdrew from social situations because she was so concerned about how her smile looked.

She didn't feel like she could even laugh at funny jokes without turning her back on the people .

So after a complete workup we sat down with Jean and talked with her about her problems. She was well aware of some of them.

That is usually the case – a person will be able to see some, and some will be totally new.

We outlined a plan for rejuvenating her smile. She accepted our recommendations and went ahead.

Jean later told us that it cost more than she had planned on, which is the case for virtually everyone. But she also said that she was glad she had done it, because she knew the effect it was going to have on her for the rest of her life.

Shortly after completing her work, she landed the promotion she had wanted. Glad for her, sad for us. It meant a move to the other coast for that new job. We congratulated her. It was yet another success for one of our patients. (Being able to help change lives like this thrills us!)

How about you? Might it be time for a little self evaluation. But before we begin, you're going to need three things: a pen to write things down, a mirror and a bright light. I'm going to ask you to examine yourself to see if there's room for improving your smile. I'm going to provide you a checklist so you can understand exactly where your smile factor stands.

So, go ahead and get your pen and go to wherever you have a mirror and a bright light. Go ahead, I'll wait.

Okay then, do you have your pen in hand? Are you in bright light? Good.

Now, all you have to do is look at your teeth in the mirror while reading through the smile checklist provided here. As you work your way down the list, simply check off each description that applies to you. Let's get started.

> **Smile Checklist**
> - Look closely at the color of your teeth. Are they dark or stained?
> - Are your teeth worn?
> - Do they have rough, jagged edges?
> - Do they look too short?
> - Are they shaped improperly or asymmetrically?
> - Do you have old fillings ugly-ing up your mouth?
> - Are there gaps between your teeth?
> - Do you have missing teeth?
> - Do your gums show too much?
> - Do your teeth look too big or too small?
> - Do you have dark fillings in the side teeth that look grey, or worse, black when you smile? This can be a little tricky. You may have to turn to the side and actually use a second mirror so you can see your side smile. This is the smile that most smile owners miss, but others see..
> - Do you have replacement teeth that look natural or are they too fake - too white or too dark? Do you have various shades of teeth so your mouth looks like a patchwork quilt?
> - Do your teeth feel uncomfortable or painful?
> - Do you struggle to chew certain foods without pain or embarrassment?

How did you do? Now what do you think about getting some cosmetic dentistry done?

What would a shot of self-confidence, sex appeal, youth and vitality do for you?

I've already told you about some of the effects of a good-looking smile. Here's another one. Pretty women and handsome men get paid an average of somewhere between 4% and 14% more than their unattractive coworkers.

Pretty big deal, huh?

Could your smile use a little updating? Maybe a bit of remodeling?

If you're like many Americans today – the answer is a resounding, "Yes." But even if it isn't, even if you don't know why you don't like your smile, you can probably be helped.

From smile disasters to simple smile enhancements, cosmetic dentistry brings new possibilities to virtually everyone.

A smile is something you just can't successfully hide. And shouldn't have to.

Coping with An Ugly Smile

If you have a mouth full of chipped, stained or jumbled teeth, life can be pretty tough. You can try to do the toothless grin with your smile clamped shut. You can always test the famous partial smile, showing just a hint of teeth but no real detail. You could even practice turning your head away when you laugh or cover your mouth with your hand.

None of these work. People notice your smile.

It's no longer necessary for you to live with the stress and strain of insecurity like this. It's holding you back, particularly today, when it can be fixed.

You know, unlike dieting or exercise, fixing your teeth is something you can do without a lot of work. You don't have to join a weight loss support group or do all kinds of uncomfortable things. You don't have to show up at exercise class at 6:00AM in the morning with a group of buff body builders or drag yourself at the end of the day to another workout class you don't want to attend.

In many cases, getting cosmetic dentistry merely involves sitting back and watching the magic unfold. As we're wont to say, you'll wonder where the ugly went.

Here's another piece of good news. The procedures really don't take very long. Often, only a few short weeks or months, depending on your situation. Sometimes only one visit!

Here are the facts. The more beautiful and alluring your smile, the more people notice you. The more they like you. The less they notice those little wrinkles and crow's feet and lines in your face. In many cases, a good-looking smile is more important than a face lift.

The power of a magnificent smile can be that dramatic. If you're thinking these benefits can't apply to you, think again. Just because you think your teeth are too messed up, it doesn't mean they are. In fact, virtually everyone can have it put right again. There's a reason. It's called the miracle of cosmetic dentistry.' We, as dentists, work with them every day. I can promise you won't be an exception.

In our society, beauty is one of those characteristics that is given a lot of credence. In fact, research shows that we automatically, without even thinking about it, assign other favorable traits like talent, kindness, honesty and intelligence to it.

What's really shocking is we make these judgments without being aware that the physical attractiveness plays a part in the process. That can be scary. Or something you can use to your advantage.

Who knows what fortunes might come into your life, without lifting a finger, if you only increase your attractor factor.

So, what makes up a pretty smile? You've probably heard the quote, "I'll know it when I see it." That's the way most people think.

They unconsciously perceive your smile and everyone else's as being attractive or unattractive depending on a number of factors.

First of all, having all of your teeth present makes a big difference. Even when a single tooth is missing it has a significant effect on how people perceive you. Can you say hillbilly anyone?

I know some people are proud of being hillbilly but they also have pretty teeth.

Second, there shouldn't be any gaps or spaces. The teeth should sit next to one another. There should also be symmetry of the teeth with your face. The middle, what we call the midline, of your upper front teeth should set between those two little ridges on your upper lip. That's called the philtrum. They should be in the midline of your face and they should be perpendicular to the floor you are standing on.

The teeth should have the right angulation. The size should match your face. Teeth too small make you look childish. Teeth too big make you look deformed.

And the color of the teeth should match your age. (Although, we will help you cheat this a little by making the teeth look like you are ten to fifteen year younger.)

Now, how light can you make the color of your teeth without looking fake? One rule of thumb is the whites of your eyes, what is known as the sclera of your eye. The brighter and whiter the sclera of your eyes, the easier it is to make teeth that are lighter in color and have them look natural.

What about the shape of teeth? Is that important? Absolutely. Each individual tooth has a specific natural shape.

And the position of your teeth makes a difference, as well.

Bad Breath and How to Solve It

If you have bad breath from time to time, welcome to life. This occurs most of the time because of the foods we eat. The second most important reason that we have bad breath is because of chronic infection of your mouth. Gum disease. Otherwise known as periodontal disease.

When you get periodontal disease, it can make your breath smell bad because of the smell created by the bacteria in your mouth. Not only can these bacteria live in your gums, they can also live on the top of your tongue. This is reason alone to clean your tongue with a toothbrush or tongue scraper.

By the way, if after brushing and flossing thoroughly and scraping your tongue, you still have chronic bad breath, you should see a dentist right away, because you probably do have gum disease. And if you don't, there may be a more serious body problem.

In our society, a big broad smile is considered beautiful. Some people have very narrow teeth arches and their smile looks narrower because of it. It needn't be this way.

What about the texture of the teeth? Texture alone can change the reflection of light. Meaning it can affect how much light is reflected back when you smile. The older we get, the smoother teeth get as a result of aging and cleaning and eating. Often times, changing the texture of the teeth can make them look more youthful.

What about your gums? Gums have an enormous effect on the appearance of teeth. In fact, gum position has its very own symmetry. (And it isn't even all the way across the smile, either.)

Gums should not be red and inflamed. In fact, red and inflamed gums indicate disease. By the way, do you have any gum disease? If your gums bleed when you brush or floss it's a problem.

What about the eruption of the teeth? Did they come all the way in? Sometimes teeth never fully erupt through the gum and get stuck short. This can make your teeth look too small and your gums too big. The correction is very straightforward.

How about wear on teeth? Worn teeth make you look older. Sadly, some people think that their upper front teeth should be even all the way across. Not so. That's a sign of aging.

The only people that have even teeth all the way across are those who've worn the teeth excessively and have never done anything about it.

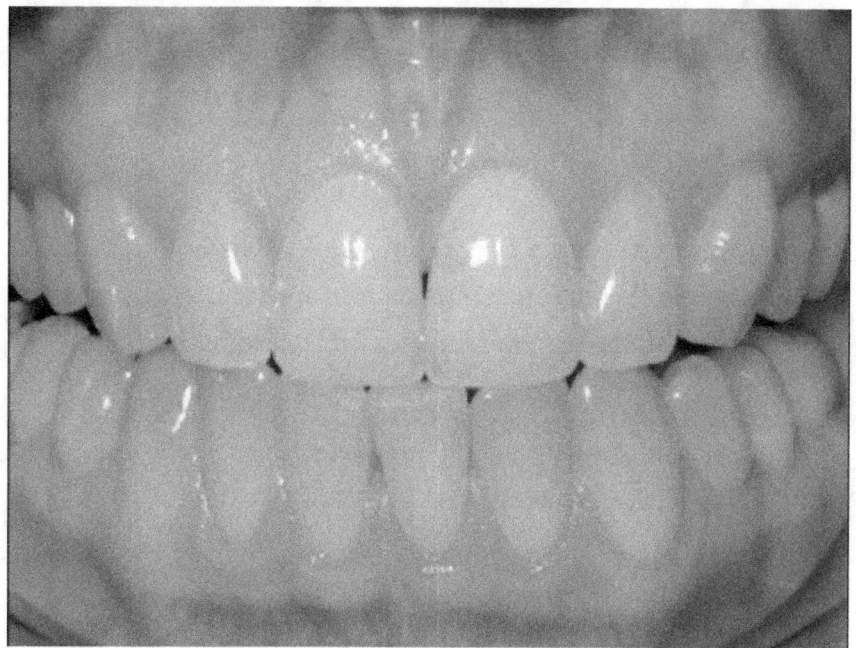

Normal tooth and gum symmetry.

The two upper front middle teeth and the two side teeth at the canines, that set underneath your eyes, should be similar length. And the teeth in between should be shorter. (Those are called the lateral incisors.)

Our rule of thumb - we like to make teeth look 10 to 15 years younger than the actual chronological age in adults older than 40.

How Much of Your Teeth Show?

How much of your teeth show? We know as you grow older your upper lip becomes longer. This causes your upper teeth to show far less. The lower lip gets more flaccid. These result from the effects of gravity on the face.

While the display of teeth shortens on the top as we grow older, the display of teeth on the lower increases because the lower lip becomes looser. And now, the lower front teeth become cosmetic teeth, because they show more.

This can make lower front teeth become as important to the smile as their upper front teeth.

If you are short, you smile will look, quite literally, foreshortened. The lower teeth become more important in appearance, because other people can see all the way into the back on their lower teeth.

And when you're tall, the upper teeth become more important as the display of teeth when smiling or talking can show the upper back teeth. So, they become pertinent to your look.

Your Face

Having a correct and properly aligned bite will also aid in optimizing one's facial appearance. Faces are meant to have certain proportions. Without a correctly balanced jaw position, one's face can look to small or disproportionate.

What about your lips? Thick lips mean that more teeth should show. If the lips are thin and the teeth are big, your smile can look a bit horsey. Lip size and tooth size should match. Big lips indicate the need for big teeth. Take a good look at Angelina Jolie as an example. Some say she has the sexiest smile of all celebrities.

Facial symmetry is important. Now, virtually no one has a perfectly symmetrical face. Still symmetry of the face is one of the unconscious ways other evaluate your looks. Having a balanced symmetrical smile is one of the ways to increase the total symmetry of the face. It is virtually impossible to have and maintain a beautiful, symmetrical face without having teeth that match.

Boomer Problems

If you were born between 1946 and 1964, you're a Baby Boomer. And as a Boomer, you had all kinds of different experiences, some good, some not so good. Today, the old-fashioned dentistry of yesteryear is gone. Good Riddance.

Here's the thing that you should realize: those fillings that you had placed when you were a kid are getting pretty old. Those old fillings could have started breaking down and leaking after all these years. One dental school study showed that 68% of those old fillings had decay under them. So what you have thought was okay, very well may not be.

Your teeth can start looking "aged and tired" way before their time, simply because of aging fillings and bite stresses. The stresses and stains of daily living can add up.

The good news is that you don't have to put up with it anymore. The advances that we've made in cosmetic dentistry and technology for dentistry have made a huge change in the way dentistry is practiced (Which we are all thankful for).

Obviously, as parents or grandparents "on the go," you need the vibrancy, look and comfort of a smile that looks as good as you want to feel, wouldn't you agree?

It seems as though that not a day goes by without some advertisement touting one skin cream or another. Skin is important to your appearance, but on the ladder of appearance, it's somewhere between third and fourth.

Your smile is number one, and your eyes are number two.

Wrinkles and Signs of Aging

If you live long enough, you're going to get wrinkles. It just goes with the package. However, a wrinkle becomes more important to your appearance when your smile doesn't look good. Wrinkles seem to become more prominent as one's smile becomes less.

You smile less when your smile doesn't look good. And therefore, the facial imperfections show more frequently. The opposite is also true. If you have a big broad smile, the wrinkles can seemingly disappear because your smile becomes the center of attention.

Smile Lines, Age, Lip Pulls and Tooth Display

The line of your smile can be broad or it can be narrow. It can be short or it can be tall. What's important is that it matches your age and it fits your face.

Smile lines that don't look right can be fixed. Sometimes the muscles around the lips will be unbalanced causing lip pulls that cause more teeth to show on one side than the other. These attachments can also change the natural display of teeth. Muscle attachments can be released to allow more teeth to show, or they can be constricted so less teeth show.

How much teeth you display when you smile is important. And things can be done so you can display more teeth to cheat your age so that you look younger.

Not Every Dentist is a Cosmetic Dentist

Well, you wouldn't know that if you read their ads or what they put on their business cards. Now, this isn't a slam against dentists. Every dentist likes to consider themselves a cosmetic dentist, but some are better than others.

Make sure that when you're looking for a cosmetic dentist, that you find one that actually is one, and not just someone who says, "I'm a cosmetic dentist."

Cosmetic dentistry is an art form and a science. And while it is not a specialty of dentistry, it does take training and an understanding of what makes a beautiful smile and pretty teeth.

Acid Reflux Disease

GERD (Gastroesophogeal Reflux Disease.)

Gastroesophageal reflux is a disease in which partially digested food and or stomach acids come up through the esophagus into the mouth. So far, we have only partial answers as to why it occurs. It can be food allergies. It can be overeating. It can be spicy food. Whatever it is, acid reflux is a very serious problem for your teeth.

Why is it so bad? The problem is the acid. Your stomach has acids that it uses to help breakdown and digest your food. This acidity is perfectly normal **within the stomach**, where is supposed to be. Your stomach is built for it. <u>Your teeth are not</u>.

Recently, I experienced a patient of mine who came in with great deal of decay. I was shocked. She was too. I inquired as to what had happened. She didn't tell me about the acid reflux. But she did tell me that her husband had been diagnosed with cancer and that she'd been very worried and hadn't been keeping her mouth as clean as she should. That didn't explain the sudden onset of severe decay. Upon further questioning, I discovered that she did have gastric reflux which explained her severe decay. The acids of her stomach were eating her teeth alive. The good news: with the correct medical management and dental care, we were able to stop the decay, manage her gastic reflux and put her smile back together again. You should see her now!

Sprucing Up Your Smile

Many people who have had a natural, good-looking smile fail to consider how they could spruce it up.

Sometimes simply whitening the teeth can make a difference. Sometimes adding a little bonding can make a difference. Sometimes just simply replacing old fillings that are dark can make a big difference.

When you check your smile out, look in the mirror. You might find yourself saying, "Hmm I wonder what it would look like if I did something about that little area. How much better would I look?"

Sprucing up your smile can be the thing that gives you a psychological boost, a "shot in the arm" and makes you feel better about yourself.

Bruxism, Worn Teeth and Clenching

It's been said that one-third of the population in North America has parafunction.

The definition of parafunction is: <u>function outside of normal</u>. This includes abnormally high force on the teeth during clenching, grinding and abnormal movements of the jaws. Most of these parafunctional events occur when you aren't conscious of them, especially during sleep. Some people have parafunction during waking hours, but few.

Parafunction causes worn teeth, broken teeth, cracked fillings, and wear of teeth before their time. It can cause teeth to get so short that they can become unattractive and even difficult to see. This doesn't happen overnight. It happens over time, usually years. Worn teeth like these make you look much older than you actually are. It can cause so much wear, that even your gums come into contact with one another!

Parafunction includes grinding and clenching your teeth, and bringing your teeth together in strange ways because you find it somehow stress relieving. Unfortunately, teeth were not built to be ground on this way. This can cause terrifically difficult headaches that won't go away, in spite of medication and treatment. Usually bite equilibrations and protective splints are needed.

Paradoxically, many of the anti-depressants that have become so frequently used are culprits in bruxism and parafunction. Some dentists believe that more than 50% of all anti-depressant users brux their teeth!

Big Problem Dentistry

If you have big dental problems you can be assured that it's going to take big solutions to fix them. Unlike simple check up dentistry with its relatively simple solutions, big problems cause geometric increases in complexity. Gum disease, replacing multiple missing teeth with dental implants, and doing cosmetic smile makeovers are all complex care. The more complex the care, the larger the fees to correct the problems. The complex care procedures require a different level of expertise, different techniques, technology, materials and lab support.

It is best if you never have to get this type of complex care. So job one is to prevent yourself from ever getting into this situation. However, if you find yourself needing this level of care, beware someone who doesn't treat it as any different than regular day to day, check up care dentistry. It really is a very different level of care. There is just too much involved.

So you need someone who has the expertise to get this type complex care work done. And if you do get in the situation, just understand that big problem dentistry fees are going to be a lot higher than those for little problem dentistry.

Snap-On Smiles

You may have seen or heard about 'Snap-On Smiles, which literally snap on to your existing teeth to change the appearance of the smile by replacing missing or stained teeth.

What's the problem with Snap-On Smiles? Well, they don't look good up close because they're bulky. They were never meant to be a long-term solution. They are a short-term solution to cosmetic problems. Using treatment like Snap-On Smiles is fine for a period of weeks or months; you will need to consider that significant problems need significant solutions for long term successful care. Snap-On Smiles is only for the short term and wear out or break or stain after a few months.

No Tooth-Preparation Porcelain Veneers

Porcelain veneers are thin sheets of porcelain designed to go over the fronts and edges of upper and lower front teeth to change the color, shape, texture or length of the teeth. These can help create a beautiful new smile for you that lights up a room.

We use them all the time. They normally require us to prepare the teeth by removing some enamel and some normal tooth structure. However, there are a small number of cases in which no tooth preparation is necessary. For instance, if there are gaps and spaces or one has small teeth, sometimes no tooth preparation is needed at all.

The mistake that can occur is to use no preparation porcelain veneers in the wrong place, when you need the teeth prepared to receive the veneers for best cosmetics, fit and bite.

Speed Dentistry

What is speed dentistry? It means getting dental care done as fast as possible. In the years past, treatment could take considerable longer. Today, with an experienced, well-trained dentist, you can get your care completed much faster. Thus the term speed dentistry. Often, procedures can be combined into a single visit instead of piece them together over multiple visits. What's more, often complete treatment can be finished on the same day.

Choosing the Right Cosmetic Dentist for You

How can you make sure you don't choose the wrong dentist?

How do you know?

Ask for proof. Ask to see before and afters of their actual patients. Ask to hear or read the testimonials of the patients they've treated. See if they have testimonials from other dentists. Ask them if it's in their comfort zone to treat cases like yours, cosmetically.

Do a little gut check of your own. Does what the dentist says seem to be trustworthy?

Check out the dentist's training. How much training has the dentist done in cosmetic dentistry? How about experience? How long has the dentist been performing cosmetic treatments?

Do you like the dentist that you're considering? You're going to have to work with them pretty extensively, so it's a good idea if you can like them and actually become friends.

Beware about basing your decision on bargains. Excellent cosmetic dentistry is virtually never a bargain. It doesn't have to be expensive. But in many cases, choosing a bargain will result in you having to do it twice. Cheap can cost twice as much as excellence from the beginning.

The Second Age of the Sweet Tooth

I find many of my patients in their 50's, 60's, 70's and 80's somehow come to the conclusion that "Ah, heck with it. I'm going to eat what I want and enjoy it." This can be dangerous thinking, no matter how attractive.

I would love to agree with them if I could. As you have probably guessed, I cannot.

The problem is many older patients take medications that dry the mouth. And with the dryness of the mouth comes less ability for your body to fight off the bacteria that cause decay and even gum disease.

Snacks before bed, including ice cream and milk, can often generate a wave of decay at the worst possible time. Milk products, in particular, promote the growth of a specific bacteria known to cause decay on the roots of the teeth. Many older patients have exposed roots on their teeth, thus putting themselves at more risk for decay.

So, beware of your own sweet tooth. It could lead to the demise of your teeth and gums. Am I saying you can't eat sweet things? No. I'm saying don't overdo it. Eat sweets in moderation and clean your mouth afterwards.

So, if you want to look your best, where do you start? Well, first things first. Earlier I gave you a self-analysis that you could do in front of your mirror. Make a list of your questions and concerns.

What bothers you about your smile?

What would you like to have happen to your smile to correct it or enhance it?

Now apply your own magic wand technique.

Ask yourself, "How would I really like to have my smile? How good do I really want it to look?"

You can use pictures of yourself when you did like your smile as a comparison.

Ask around. Most people will go on the Internet and do a bit of research. Ask for a consultation to discuss your cosmetic needs. Meet the dentist. Learn what the dentist has to say and then expect to have a clinical exam of the diagnostic records made. These can range from a few dollars to up to $1,000 or more, depending upon your condition.

Then you should have a consultation. At your consultation ask for what I call proof of competence. Ask nicely, of course, but do ask. Ask to see cases of other patients.

You should work to become a partner in the process. Unlike much of healthcare where you just sit there or lay there, dentistry is done *with* you. It is a partnership. The better a partner you are, the faster, easier and better it goes.

A dentist is going to be largely incapable of overcoming something you will not do.

You have to be a partner in the process to make it successful, which means home care, diet and regular professional maintenance.

Ask if there are any warranties or guarantees. Although we can't guarantee everything – you are a living, breathing, changing entity - most of the best dentists will stand behind what they do and correct problems.

Now I'm going to give you what I call the counterintuitive stroke of genius. The vast majority of dentists feel, in general, under-appreciated.

Now, I'm not asking you to feel sorry for dentists. But I am telling you something that will help you get the best work of the best dentists. Show your appreciation. Say thank you early and often. Make a big deal of big results. Your dentist doesn't hear it often. Your appreciation works magic on the relationship, and ultimately the care you receive. Refer friends and family and your dentist will become your greatest ally.

More Than Looks

Cosmetic procedures are more than just about looks. They also require functionality, gum health, and the correct bite. Building them to last also requires an understanding of the source of your problems. Without these things, cosmetic dentistry is more likely to fail.

So, let's talk about the different types of cosmetic procedures that are available, who's a candidate for them and if they're appropriate for you.

The first and easiest are bleaching and whitening. Millions of people have had their teeth whitened by bleaching. This has become a very common procedure, and for good reason.

For those with little or no other dental problems, bleaching to whiten the teeth is one of the most successful cosmetic procedures that can be done. The results can be spectacular.

However, bleaching the teeth is not without problems. Not all teeth bleach the same. Over the counter brands are not as strong as the prescription strength ones a good dentist can use. Not all teeth whiten the same. If your teeth are yellowy, they bleach more easily. If they are gray, brown or blue, they are harder to bleach.

Virtually everyone can have natural tooth structure whitened. However, old fillings, porcelain, and old restorations do not whiten.

What happens when you whiten your teeth? You're removing the extrinsic stains from a lifetime of food, dark liquids, candy, colas and wine. For smokers, the tars and nicotine leave dark brown and yellow stains that just won't brush off. Bleaching actually opens up little teeny pores inside the crystalline structure of teeth and removes the pigments from it so the teeth look whiter.

Virtually everyone with natural teeth, no matter how dark, can have their teeth whitened these days.

There are three types of bleaching. There is in-office power bleaching using dentist provided materials and technology. This one's the most effective. The fees for this can range from 500 dollars on the low side up to 2,000 dollars or more for very darkly stained teeth caused by tetracycline staining. Most people are in the lower end of that range.

The second involves having custom trays made that you use overnight or during the day at home. These cost somewhat less. But for many people, the inconvenience and additional time required make it less popular. This method can take weeks longer to be successful.

The third way involves using the over the counter products. A few of these over the counter products can work pretty well in selected cases. However, many also have not been FDA approved and have only varying degrees of success. It can be very hard to get this method of teeth whitening correct. We get lots of people who tried to use these products on their own finally give up and come to us to get it done professionally.

Cosmetic Contouring

Cosmetic contouring is artfully reshaping the length, width, edges and thickness of your teeth so they look better. It's helpful for teeth that are slightly turned, slightly too long or misshaped.

Cosmetic contouring helps individualize the teeth, and can make some look less bucky or less turned. Although there are limitations to what cosmetic contouring can do, it is probably the most underused of all parts of cosmetic dentistry.

Bonding

Bonding is the application of tooth-colored plastics to your teeth using a technique that bonds the life-like material to the tooth itself. It has many advantages. Its most frequent use is to repair cavities and replace decayed tooth structure.

When used specifically for changing the appearance of teeth, it can help close small spaces and gaps. It can be used to lengthen or widen teeth.

Bonding has now been around and has been used successful since the 1970's. However, there are problems with bonding. It can stain and discolor. It can break. It can chip and crack. The variance in the ability of the dentist to bond has a huge effect on this long-term success of bonding. Even more, how a particular patient functions against the bonding has an even bigger effect on long term success of it. Some people are just "rough" on their teeth. Some put excessive forces against the bonding by gnawing on bones or using their teeth to open packages. There are hundreds of ways to break a bonded tooth. This is why many dentists prefer bonding stronger materials to the teeth than plastic. They have learned from experience that too many patients inadvertently treat bonded teeth as if they need no special care.

Even more important to the long term success of bonding is an individual's own dental hygiene. Omitted hygiene or poor hygiene dooms any dentistry, including bonding, to an early demise.

When used properly, bonding is one of the most effective ways to repair or enhance the look of the teeth.

Bonding, by the way, is also being used now to cement or attach crowns. It can be used to eliminate the black, dark fillings in the back teeth. Many patients appreciate the look of white back teeth when talking or laughing.

Caution: If Your Teeth Are Worn

For many people looking to correct excessively worn teeth, cosmetic dentistry can be a real bonanza… when it is done as part of a total plan that includes solving why you wore down your teeth in the first place!

Cosmetic procedures can and should be used to help correct bite issues. If your bite is off, your teeth will wear excessively. As your teeth wear, they look worse. Often the wear propagates more wear. This can be a vicious cycle. Putting it all back together again is never as simple as just adding material to the teeth to make the size and shape more cosmetically pleasing. It takes a lot more than that. Treating complex bite issues is among the most challenging of all parts of dentistry! Not only must the cosmetic procedures be done well, the entire chewing mechanism and bite function must be addressed. To the average person who knows nothing of this complexity, it can seem like a whole lot of dentistry to correct what he or she thought would be pretty simple. The

Pregnancy and Dental Care

If you are considering becoming pregnant, make sure your teeth are in good health before you get pregnant. And if you're already pregnant do as much as you can to care for them. You are likely to have gums that are more puffy, even red, because of hormonal changes associated with your pregnancy.

However, with good brushing and flossing that doesn't have to be the case. If you do have that problem during your pregnancy, you should see a dentist to have some basic hygiene care done to remove the causes of the inflammation.

If you have significant dental problems, especially gum disease problems, you can put yourself at risk of having a low birth weight baby and/ or pre-mature birth. Both of these put you and your baby at significant risk! While not ideal, if you have dental problems during pregnancy, you should get them treated to prevent the infections that can wreak havoc with you and your baby.

work must be integrated together to not only look good but also function properly while protecting against future excessive wear. Usually protective plastic appliances must be made for nighttime wear to protect against the renewal of excessive wear habits.

Porcelain Veneers

The television shows that demonstrated extreme smile makeovers changed the way many people think about dental care – and that is a good thing. For millions, it was the first time that they really understood the power of having a beautiful smile.

One of the procedures done to help create those smiles is porcelain veneers.

Veneering literally means removing a portion of a tooth and placing a veneer of porcelain over the top and over the edge of the teeth, bonding them into place to change the shape or color or position or texture.

It can be a very successful, conservative procedure, although it doesn't answer all problems.

Veneering gives a very natural look and is something which every cosmetic dentist worth his salt as a cosmetic dentist does on a regular basis.

What about dental crowns? Well, crowns always used to be made of metal. Then came metal and plastic versions. But the plastic wore out. Then they were made of metal and porcelain. But the metal could show.

Today there are porcelain and metal crowns where the metal doesn't show at all. We also have complete porcelain crowns made of high strength ceramics. There's a whole range of these ceramics for different purposes that allow light to show through the teeth just like natural teeth do.

Veneers used well and in the right situations can utterly transform the way your smile looks. Cosmetic crowns made of esthetic materials can give higher strength where needed. Choosing what is right for you is a decision for you and your dentist.

Plastic Surgery for Your Gums

Your gum tissue has its own form, texture, color, shape and position. Usually these factors are dictated by the teeth, but often due to inflammation, tooth loss, abnormal position of teeth or gum recession, the gum can move into positions too high or too low on the teeth. Sometimes, the tissue itself will lose the attachment to the root making the tooth more liable for infection and breakdown. Asymmetries of gum position can result from mismatched bites and over or under-erupted teeth. When the gums aren't "right" it is nigh on impossible to give the teeth the right look.

Plastic surgery for your gums can solve all these problems and more. We can actively intervene to move your gums using periodontal plastic surgery techniques. These procedures can reposition gum tissue around your teeth to create symmetry, gain new attachment of tissue and show the right gum length on each tooth.

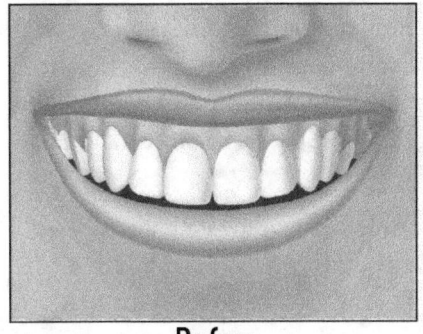
Before

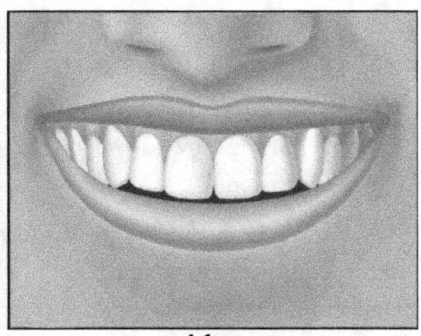
After

Invisalign

Invisalign uses clear trays that have pressures built into them to move teeth. These can successfully help change teeth positions inside an arch.

Invisalign may do a poor job of coordinating the upper arch to the lower arch if your malocclusion is severe. Which means it can throw off your bite in the process of straightening your smile.

However, Invisalign does have some advantages. It's virtually invisible. There are no brackets and wires. You can go ahead with normal activities. In the right situation, it can be a rear perfect solution.

Still, a slight disadvantage of Invisalign is that it might cost more than regular orthodontics and it's uncommon to get the results you can with conventional orthodontic treatment if your teeth are severely maligned.

The biggest mistake you can make is to do nothing about your dental problems. Doing so almost always makes problems worse.

Likewise, I often see people only treat the appearance of their teeth without considering the health of their teeth. They may have a treatment that improves the look of teeth without taking care of function.

This takes its toll, and can eventually factor into early death. If a person has significant periodontal disease, it can cause infections that overwhelm the body without you knowing about it.

Another mistake people make is not finding the right expert for their situation. You need someone with competence to do the kind of work you need. The more complex the work, the more you need an expert.

Another mistake is making decision based solely on economics. Cheap may cost you far more in the long run.

For example, when you're doing cosmetic dentistry, the artisans that create the porcelain veneers and crowns naturally have to take more time to create them. So, a cosmetic crown can cost the dentist four to ten times what a normal crown would. That's got to be reflected in the fees that are charged to you.

A mistake that other people make is not understanding their choices. It's important for you to understand what choices you have and to make an informed decision about what cosmetic dentistry can do for you.

For some people, a gummy smile can be embarrassing. With these techniques, we can often change the gummy look into the just right look, where the amount of tooth that shows is enlarged while the gum is decreased. On the other hand, the situation can be reversed – not enough gum shows. If this is the case, procedures can be done to release muscles that bind your lips to cover too much of your teeth.

A frequent condition for many people is that their teeth look too short. Often this is caused by an alteration in the way the teeth erupt. Sometimes all that is needed is to uncover what is there. The procedures can be used to reveal the teeth hiding underneath excessive gums. Sometimes this involves removing just soft tissue, and the more likely scenario is the need to re-shape bone and soft tissue that cover the teeth. It sounds more difficult for you that it actually is. Recovery is rapid and the results are tremendous.

I've had more than one patient come to me and ask me for porcelain veneers on their front teeth so they'll look better.

After I look at their smiles, I often find that the problem is not that their teeth don't look good. It's their gums are inappropriately positioned so they don't display enough teeth. For these people, we can redesign the smile with periodontal plastic surgery that reveals more teeth so their smile looks great.

Smile Enhancement

Covering Tooth Roots

Today, we're able to do a version of oral plastic surgery to improve the appearance of the gums, actually rebuild missing soft tissue that attaches to the teeth.

More uses of Additive Periodontal Surgery:

- Create gum symmetry so the teeth have an enhanced pleasing look.

- Add tissue to cover tooth roots to stop more recession and bone loss and improve the looks of teeth. Moreover, this can stop tooth sensitivity.

- Build up missing gum tissue to balance the appearance with the other teeth.

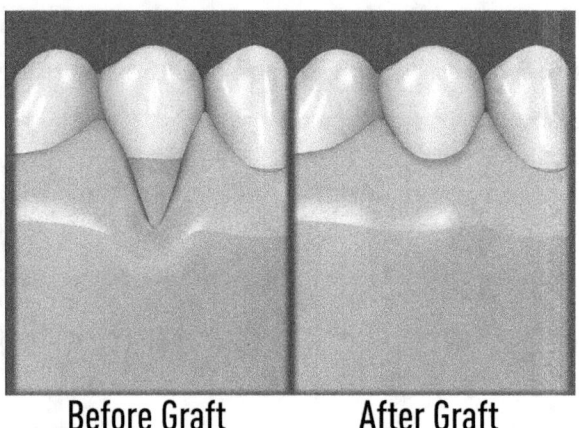

Before Graft   **After Graft**

- Graft bone to rebuild and/or replace missing bone structure. (This has some limitations.)

New technology includes using tissue substitutes for soft tissue grafting, special proteins to stimulate bone growth and growth factor concentrates from your own blood.

The Dark Tooth

If you have a single dark tooth in the front, typically it has had some injury that caused the nerve to break down or possibly even die. When this happens, the living tissue inside the root dies, breaks down and discolors. The result is a tooth that looks dark. It can often stand out in someone's smile like a sore thumb. The thing about a sore thumb is that you can hide it. Your dark tooth is there for all to see.

Often all that's required to fix it is root canal therapy to remove the darkened contents from inside the root. Then a bleach is placed inside that root to bleach out the remaining darkness to have it match the other color of the teeth. It is not expected to get a perfect match, but it will be better than the contrast that was there before.

Who would have ever thought that root canal therapy would be a cosmetic procedure?

Replacing Missing Teeth

There are four technologies to replace missing teeth these days. I'll go through them.

Number one is dental implants. Dental implants have become the premier method of replacing missing teeth. And for good reason. I'll explain.

The first thing to understand is that replacing missing teeth should happen, because the missing tooth that is not replaced has effects that cascade into your entire smile. It can cause gaps to form, decrease chewing ability, increase gum disease and actually cause loss of other teeth.

So, it's no small matter to leave a missing tooth unreplaced. Teeth will invariably move around into positions where you don't want them.

A dental implant helps prevent that from occurring.

On the other hand, conventional dental bridges use crowns on adjacent teeth with a pontic – the false tooth-in between. Generally

What's New?

What's new in dentistry?

- All ceramic restorations that reflect light like natural teeth.

- Surgical techniques to help rebuild gums and bone.

- Human growth factors taken from your body and then concentrated. This is used in surgical situations to speed healing, to increase comfort and improve results.

- Dental implants to replace missing teeth. Dental implants are the next best thing to a natural healthy tooth.

- Bonding technology to dental restorations last longer, look better and seal better.

- Advancements in the science of color, understanding what makes color and how we can apply it to dental materials so your teeth look as natural as possible.

- Deeper understanding of the biology of function, mechanics and cosmetics and the relationships these have on having a successful smile, oral health and functional teeth.

- We have a better understanding of the effects that your smile and teeth have on you, your sense of wholeness, your sense of wellbeing, your sense of self-worthiness and how others treat you because of your looks. This has been a real advance we didn't know previously. We empirically knew before, now studies prove it to us.

- Real alternatives to the standard therapy of the past: tooth removal "Just take it out, Doc," is not the preferred, first solution to dental problems.

- We understand the relationship a tooth has to your health. And for that reason, dentistry has actually become more important, not less, in modern day health care.

these are made of porcelain and metal to give a nice look and to have durability.

Think of a dental bridge like a bridge across a highway or river. At each end there is an abutment structure that the bridge holds onto. That's what the adjacent teeth do in a dental bridge.

In the middle is the pontoon or pontic that replaces the missing teeth. Bridge work has a good success rate and might be the most appropriate methodology for replacing missing teeth.

Unfortunately some dentists are continuing to use dental bridges work dental implants would be a better choice. Make sure, if you're having a missing tooth replaced, that you're having it replaced the best way possible. The best replacement will vary from individual to individual based upon the condition of the teeth that are going to be part of the bridge and how much bone is available for a dental implant.

A removable partial denture is a replacement tooth that fits on a framework of either gum colored plastic or metal that hooks around the teeth.

Beware the use of partial dentures that are all gum colored plastic. Why? These are useful as temporary solutions only. This type of removable partial denture has no support from the teeth at all. It rests only on the gums. These types of partial dentures will invariably cause a great deal

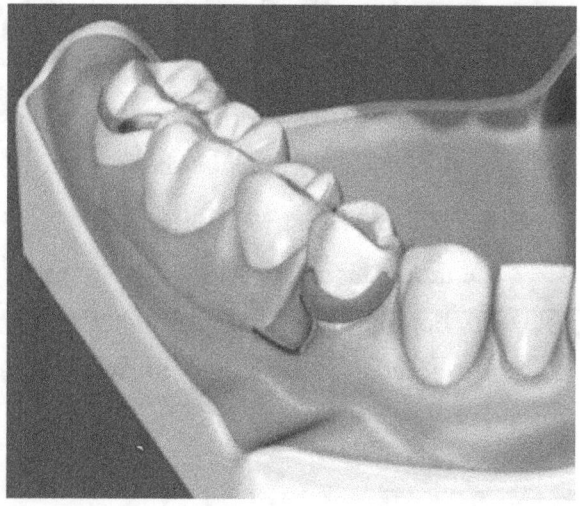

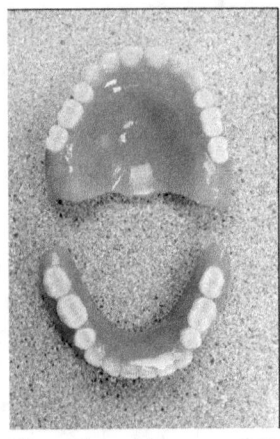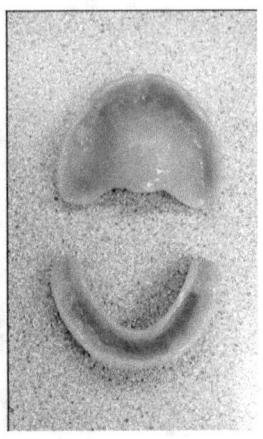

of bone loss where the pressure exists, particularly on the top of the ridge of a jaw. These all plastic partials have various names including the name flipper. This name is used when the removable partial denture replaces just 1 to 3 teeth. They are called flippers because they flip in and out. These are not a really successful methodology to use for a long term solution. These are transitional answers and short-term solutions. Some patients mistakenly think that because it "looks pretty good" that it's functioning well. Not true.

A better removable partial denture is a metal framework partial denture that distributes force on the remaining teeth and protects the gums from excessive pressure that would cause the bone loss.

There is a special bone that surrounds each tooth called alveolar bone. Alveolar bone begins to melt away when teeth are removed. The good news is that cosmetic implants maintain that alveolar bone and help maintain bone in general.

Removable partial dentures and complete removable dentures do not protect like this. They put pressure on the bone that invariably causes the compression that erodes the bone in both height and width.

The more height and width lost, the less comfortable the removable teeth become and the more difficult they are to use (and the more difficult it becomes to use dental implants because of the loss of bone).

Summary

A new smile can mean many things. It can mean greater self-confidence. It can mean a romance renewed or a romance began. It can mean a new job promotion. It can mean more money in your pocket over time. It can mean feeling better about you. It can give you a greater ability to communicate persuasively with others.

It really is very much a personal investment and it has benefits on many, many levels. There's no reason to live with embarrassment from your teeth, or the insecurity of never knowing when the next toothache could strike.

It isn't necessary to live this way anymore. Even if your situation feels hopeless, it can be improved. We have done for thousands of others; we can do it for you.

You already know your smile is one of the first things that people notice about you. Don't let an unattractive one sabotage your dreams for another minute. You can enjoy a brighter future and increase confidence. All of this is possible for you. Wouldn't it make sense to take the first step?

Complete dentures, also called plates or false teeth, are quite literally oral wigs. These are not the best solution. For some people, these are the only solution. If it can be avoided you're wise to do so.

I've had patients say. "Well, I want to get complete dentures because I don't want any more trouble with my teeth." Unfortunately they don't realize that all they're doing is creating more trouble for the future. True, there are no more teeth, but having complete dentures creates whole new, worse set of problems. You lose chewing ability and bone when you have dentures. And generally, your teeth just don't look as good when you have complete dentures.

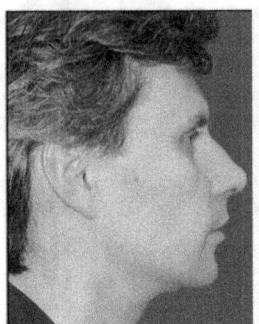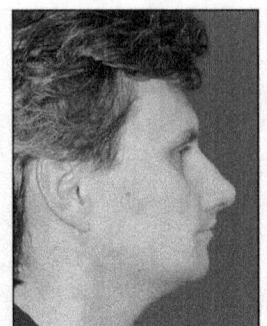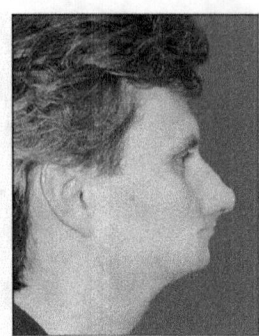

Facial Atrophy Over Time with Loss of Teeth

Replacing missing tissue and bone

Today's modern dentistry now has the ability to replace missing tissue and bone. Today we can grow back what is missing by grafting hard or soft tissue back where it belongs.

While there limits to what can be accomplished with this technique, it's now part of what we do on a regular basis. We often transplant bone or gum tissue from one part of the mouth to the place where it's deficient.

When a person has worn complete dentures for many years, it can result in an enormous loss of bone. Now we take bone from the tibia or the hip to rebuild the upper and lower jaw. For dental cripples, these procedures can make a huge difference in their lives.

Once the grafts are in place, it is important to use dental implants to help maintain that bone. Why? Because if you transplant this bone or tissue to the missing area and it does not have the stimulation that an implant can provide, the newly transplanted bone or tissue will melt away, too!

Orthognathic Surgery

Another cosmetic procedure is called orthognathic surgery. Literally, this means changing the positions of the upper and/or lower jaw so they fit the face better.

The results can be dramatic..

The downside is that it is expensive and can have complications. The upside is that it can be completed in one surgery.

Often orthognathic surgery requires orthodontic treatment in combination to reposition the teeth to get the bite right prior to moving the upper and lower jaw. I frequently send patients to have it done because I think it's in their best interest. What is important is to have an orthodontist and oral surgeon who are accustomed to working together to create your final result. While orthodontics can move teeth into specific locations, orthognathic surgery moves entire sections of teeth along with the bone.

What some people don't realize is that orthodontics is more than just about having the teeth look good. Done well, it aligns the teeth and improves function.

Orthodontics

More and more adults are using orthodontics to improve the alignment and position of the teeth. For some adults, this can save them tens of thousands of dollars by simply moving teeth where they belong, getting rid of gaps and spaces.

For others, the orthodontics will just simply take too long to get done. And therefore, they have other procedures done, including crown and bridgework, veneers and implants to correct the problems.

I generally advise the majority of my patients that orthodontics is the first treatment that should be considered to solve significant dental problems where it is appropriate. If you have lots of existing dental work, it is often simpler to use restorative dentistry to correct the problems. Other situations benefit from a combined approach of orthodontics plus the use of porcelain veneers, dental implants and smile design.

For some adults, orthodontics is virtually required to really correct what's wrong. You should include it among the possible methods to get your dental problems corrected.

A Big Mistake

A big mistake is letting the time needed to treat become the deterrent to treatment. For most people with significant cosmetic problems, it took years, even their lifetime to get in that condition. Sometimes it can take months or even a couple of years to get it fixed. Not a bad amount of time to get something fixed if the problem's been around a long time. Wouldn't you agree?

So, be careful of letting time be a deterrent to care. If it's going to take a couple of years, my question to you is this: if you didn't have it done and a couple years pass, it's not really any different, is it?

Another mistake is failing to understand that the more involved the work, the more it will cost and the more you need an expert who not only understands it all but can do it all and see it through.

This is probably the result of people not understanding the different facets of dentistry. What most people understand is what I call check-up dentistry. That is the normal maintenance that helps people keep their teeth and health maintained.

Cosmetic dentistry and complex dentistry require a different level of care because it's far more involved.

Another mistake that people make is ignoring their teeth. The statement: ignore your teeth and they'll go away, is true if you wait long enough. Even if you've made mistakes in the past that doesn't mean you can't take responsibility now and get things fixed like they should be.

What about partial treatment? You know, partial treatment means getting treatment that answers the problem a little bit. What's the problem with partial treatment? The problem with partial treatment is you get a partial answer.

And usually the partial answer will not be enough to get the long-term solution.

What about staging treatment in segments over time? Yes, this can work. What is important to realize is that if the bite has to change or that you have significant needs, staging treatment has many limitations. What part of the problem do you want us leave?.

The last among these mistakes is what I call Band-Aid and scotch tape dentistry. That is giving a solution that only has an appearance advantage but no other advantage at all.

You know, scotch tape falls apart pretty easily and a Band-Aid's good for a few days. When you get this kind of dentistry done you're going to get that kind of result for your teeth.

Dental Do's and Don'ts

Don't use your teeth to open a bottle or a wrapper. Using your teeth like this can cause them to break or chip needlessly. This is a very frequent reason I see emergency patients in my office.

Don't chew sugared gum or lollipops all day long to fight a breath problem. If you're going to do this make sure they're sugar free. Any substance that has sugar in it that will bathe your teeth in it over an extended period of time, that's sure to cause significant cavities The preferred sugarless sweetener is xylitol, which is a natural sweetener that's safe for your teeth. We also find it helps fight dental plaque, believe it or not.

Avoid really abrasive toothpaste. While this may give you the sense that you're getting your teeth their whitest, it also takes part of the enamel with it. Don't do it.

Avoid biting your nails, it causes excessive wear on your teeth. This is especially true when you've had cosmetic dentistry done. You can cause dental work to break or chip.

If you have a retainer make sure you wear it. Not wearing your retainer after you've had braces is almost sure to allow teeth to revert to their former positions.

Avoid going to a bargain dental place. You're going to get what you pay for. And we've seen too many patients who've come to us begging for us to fix the bargain care. Now the person has to pay for it twice.

Don't use somebody else's toothbrush. The bacteria laden in that toothbrush can give you disease. I suggest that you keep the following in mind. If you have a family member, a loved one, a spouse who has gum disease, understand that it's possible for them to pass it onto you. While this passing on is not widely understood, it just makes sense that if you're sharing foods and glasses or liquids with one another, that you can get your spouse's bugs. You don't want to do this. This is the reason for you to insist that the ones you love and care about are also maintaining high levels of dental health.

Avoid piercings in your tongue. We've seen some very wicked infections with tongue piercings. They also can cause you to chip teeth. You can even swallow these things. These tongue piercings can also cause damage to the teeth themselves. It is not a pretty thing.

Don't go to bed without brushing and flossing. The food products that you have on your teeth can set there all night long, wreaking havoc. So, if you have a peanut butter and jelly sandwich before you to go bed, make sure you brush and get that peanut butter and jelly off your teeth. If you're going to have a glass of milk before bed, at least rinse your mouth and preferably brush your teeth after that glass of warm milk. Ice cream before bed is the same: rinse and clean.

The older you are the more susceptible you are to a bacterium that just loves dairy products, lactobacillus, which can cause decay in the tooth roots of your teeth.

Avoid using over the counter whitening products; they're unpredictable. You don't know what you're going to get. You're much better off having a professional help you whiten your teeth.

Help your child, if he or she is sucking a finger or digit, not to do that. After about age three the damage that can be caused by sucking on a thumb or a finger can be significant in the development of the jaws and the position of the teeth. Make sure your dentist helps you manage this noxious habit.

If you smoke, understand that you're making your ability to heal that much more difficult. You're going to stain your teeth. And frankly, the substances in the smoke inhibit the body's own ability to heal. It inhibits collagen synthesis, which is the basic building block of soft tissue and bone.

Oh, by the way, just as a favor to the dentist, when you show up in the dental office make sure you've brushed and flossed. It just makes good sense. Plus there's no reason to be embarrassed by the things the dentist could pick off your teeth.

Don't send a child to bed with a bottle of soft drinks, milk or juices because these can cause something called baby bottle decay. Baby bottle decay cases can cause pretty significant trauma to a small child and can lead to painful memories lasting well into adulthood. Not a good idea.

Mary's Story

Mary came to us more than a bit bedraggled. She wasn't looking good at all. She wasn't even dressing nicely. She wouldn't smile to let us take pictures as part of our evaluation, which is a normal part of the process we use in diagnosing cases like hers.

Mary was separated and just three weeks from final divorce decree. She said to us, "Look I know my mouth is a mess. In fact, I know it's a disaster. I wish I'd taken better care of it, but I've spent most of life taking care of my husband and taking care of our children, making sure they had all they needed. I figure my time is now. Can you help me?"

Our heart went out to Mary. We're going to actually help set her back on her life's course where she belongs. She knew it and so did we. Mary told us she found us almost by luck. Serendipity plays its role again. She knew she needed a dentist, but didn't know where to look and was asking around and someone mentioned our name. Then she thought she'd do a search and went online and found us on the web. She proudly told us she had read every page about what we do and how we do it.

So when we sat down to talk to Mary at her consultation about what was going to be involved, she had all the normal questions. How long is it going to take? How much is it going to cost? What result can I predict I'm going to get when I get done? We answered her questions.

When we told her the fee involved she went quiet a moment. "Well, that's a lot more than I expected it to be."

We find that most patients experience this same thing. They have no idea what it costs when they have big problems like Mary had. It requires dentistry at a level two notches or more above regular general dentistry. Mary wisely decided it was in her best interest.

She said, "You know, I'm not going to tell my friends about this; and I'm not going to discuss it with my family because this is for me. What do they know about my problems and what it's going to mean for me to get my teeth fixed? They don't have my problems so they can't know."

Mary knew the answer.

Today, Mary has a beautiful smile and she's remarried. She told us she's so much happier being married this time around.

You see life throws us all types of curves. Mary made her problem into an opportunity and now has the marriage that she always wished she'd have. Was it because of her smile? Well, it certainly was attractive enough to get somebody interested in a big way!

Mary comes back to see us on a regular basis. She's one of our shining success stories. Mary decided not to listen to family and friends, in fact wouldn't even entertain the idea of doing so. She made her own wise decision.

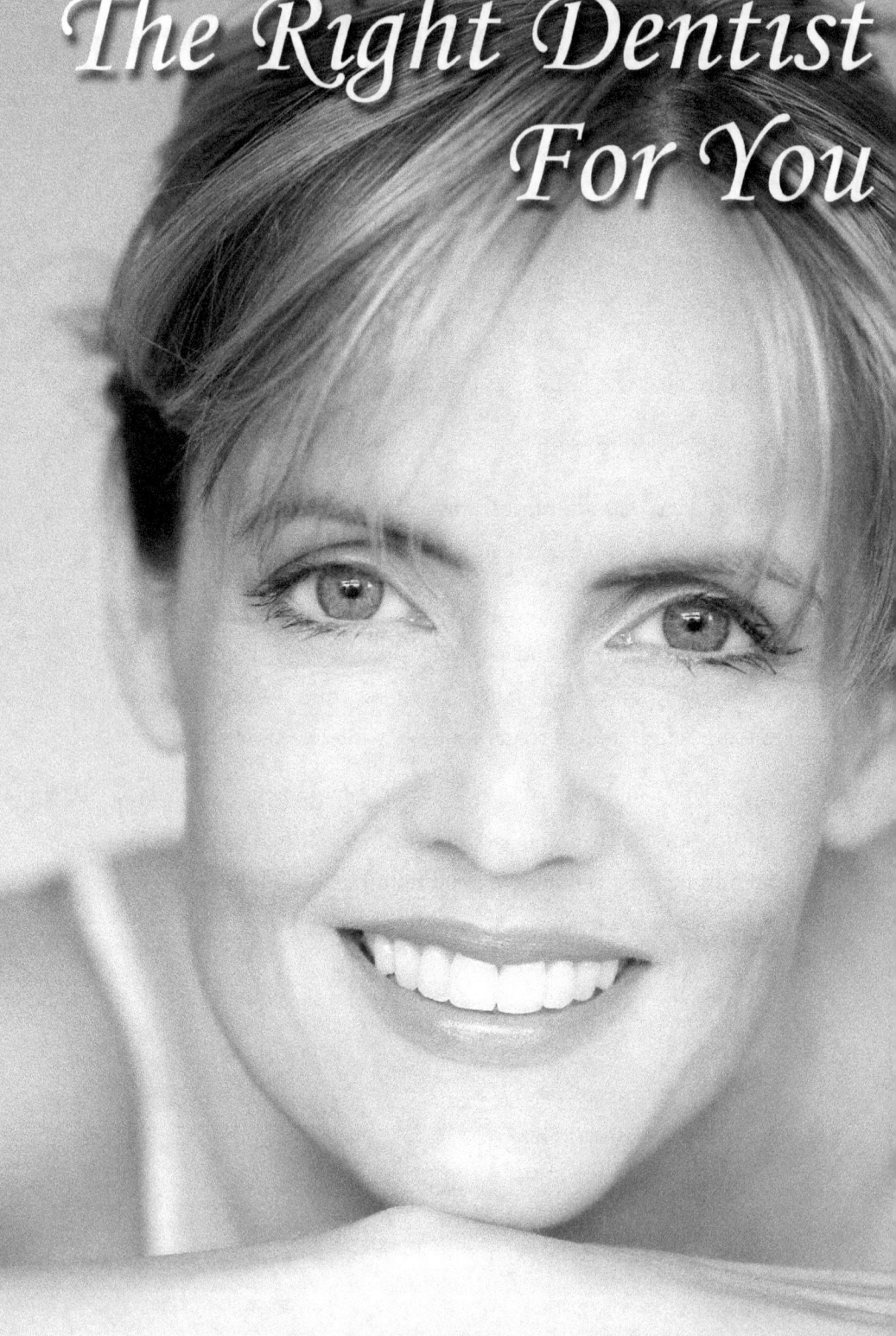

The Right Dentist For You

CHAPTER 14
The Right Dentist For You

It's a tale of two patients.

Betty, a very nice person, had been coming to us intermittently for years usually for emergencies and an occasional cleaning. Slowly, over time, her mouth had degraded, teeth had yellowed, and fillings that needed to be replaced had darkened. Missing teeth had gone unreplaced. Her bite worsened. And now she was beginning to experience jaw pain.

She told me that she had been recently diagnosed as being diabetic and her gum condition was bad. Her gums bled easily and she had chronic bad breath that wouldn't go away.

In spite of all our efforts to get Betty to do something about her teeth, she hadn't. And sadly, she never did.

Sometime after this particular visit, Betty was diagnosed with pancreatic cancer and died. What people don't know is, is if you have periodontal disease the chances of you having cancer increases.

Debbie, on the other hand, had come to us on a referral from another patient and was in a lot of trouble. She was very candid in her description of her condition. And she understood that the problem had started with her.

She also knew that she was going to have to do a lot and pay a lot to get things fixed. The good news for Debbie is that she did all that work. She did her regular maintenance. She did her home care. She did what she needed to maintain her oral health.

These many years later, Debbie now has six grandchildren and enjoys her life very much. For us that's been a stunning success. We want you to have that too.

You know, dentists and patients have two distinctly different points of view. If you mention the word dentist to the average person, most will respond negatively.

If you ask that same person about their smile or their teeth, they generally have a positive view.

To say that dentists aren't aware of this is putting one's head in the sand. Understand the dentist's dilemma: they work in a small dark, wet hole that moves, very limited access, and a tongue that has something to say about the dentist being there. And the dentist is supposed to make conditions better with treatments that last. This is all done with the precision of a Swiss watch, while tending to the emotional needs of the patient.

The patient's perspective is, "I get to open my mouth so the dentist can get in there and I get poked on, sometimes with sharp instruments. Sometimes I've had pain I didn't predict and it's uncomfortable. I get to pay money to get all this done." That's not a pretty picture either.

People know less about dentistry than any other health profession. They should know more, which is the reason for this book.

Usually geographic location is not the best way to choose the dentist. Why? Because it's the luck of the draw. Yet 80% of all people do choose based upon geographic location alone.

If we're looking for good care from a good dentist, you might get lucky and you might not.

Check to see what the atmosphere is like in their office. Does it feel right to you? Does it look right? Do they appear to be up to date?

Do they have technology that makes sense in today's world? Do you want a dentist who's outgoing or someone who remains quiet? Do you want a teacher and explainer or do you want to lay there and have your work done with as little communication as possible?

It's important for everybody to understand each other: the dentist and the patient and the staff. Some people make the mistake of withholding information because they don't trust dentists or dentistry. That can create serious problems for you. What you withhold may impact you very negatively.

A good dentist will talk you out of care that's not right for you. At the same time, they will proactively work to move you to choose the right choices for you.

So, how can you find a trusted dental advisor, a good dentist to help you?

Among other things:

- Call and talk to their office.
- Talk to their staff.
- Take a tour of their practice.
- Listen to what their patients have to say.
- Listen to what other dentists have to say about them.
- Interview the dentist, get your questions answered.
- Check your own instinctive gut reaction.
- Are you comfortable with them?
- Does your personality match up well so that you can get along well?
- Does the facility of the practice match what you think it should be?
- Does the dentist show a passion for the field?
- How much training does the dentist have?
- How many years of experience?

They will communicate with you. They'll try to make you a friend just as you should try to make a friend of them.

As a patient you have certain rights.

You have rights to good care. You have rights to explanations of care. You have the right to fairness in fee. You have a right to good personal care and treatment. You have the right to be remembered for who you are and for follow up. You have the right to get care that's tailored to you. And you have the right to have as positive a dental experience as possible.

If you want to be an outstanding patient then you have a responsibility, as well. This responsibility is to help the dentist be as successful as possible with you and other patients, to speak up when you see something that's not quite right and to tell them honestly what's going on.

You should communicate even when it's inconvenient to do so, which may mean picking up the phone and calling the dentist and let them know something that happened positively or negatively.

Dentistry is far more interactive than other areas of health care. It happens more frequently. And for this reason, it is necessary that you have a dentist that you like, enjoy and that you know does good work for you.

If the dentist makes you a promise that you doubt anyone can keep, beware. When you ask for success rates, understand they're probably going to talk to you in percentages and likelihoods and possibilities.

Look for a dentist who is involved in continuing training, who trains others or takes a lot of training on their own. If they've written articles or books, so much the better.

Are they available when you need them around?

Choosing a good dentist and having a good dental relationship is imperative for having dental health for your lifetime. With what we know, it is critical that you make good choices.

If you don't feel like you've made a good choice, find someone you can trust and feel comfortable with. And then tell them all they need to know, do all you need to do and you'll have a gorgeous smile that helps you live your best life.

Bill's Story

A quick story. I had a patient named Bill. He was a recent divorcee, 52-years old, and had a whale of a problem. His teeth were a mess. He knew they were a mess and he knew that he had to get them fixed. Bill confided in me that he wasn't sure that his smile hadn't led to part of his divorce. But now he knew that he had to do something about it.

He also knew that it was going to take a bite out of his financial backside to get it fixed. We met with Bill. We examined him. We came to understand his problems and what he wanted to have. Bill, you see, had been denying himself care for many, many years. He'd helped his children get through private school, get through college and now his wife unfortunately had decided to take off with another man.

Bill could have been bitter. But he chose to do something positive with himself. So he became a patient in our office and we began our process. After some many months, and what many would call a small fortune, Bill is now smiling again. And he's not smiling a little bit, he's got this big, bright, knock 'em out-of-the-stadium smile that anybody would die to have.

You know it's the kind of smile you get to see on the extreme makeovers; it's that kind of result. Well, as you might guess, Bill, after his divorce was devastated. He wasn't doing well emotionally. In fact, he'd become more than a little bit withdrawn because his teeth were so bad and he didn't have the regular support mechanisms he'd had before. He got laid off in his job. Things weren't looking very good.

After his makeover, Bill not only has found a new job, but has been promoted into a vice-president's position making a salary twice what he used to have. Was it because of his smile? We'd like to think so. In reality, Bill had a lot on the ball anyway. He had been knocked down by life and was hugely disappointed in the marriage he had counted on. Bill's now back. Bill didn't listen to the little voices that said he couldn't afford it; that said it wasn't the right time to do it. In fact, Bill saved his own life emotionally and financially by choosing to actively cause what he wanted in life.

What we know is that Bill not only saved his life right now; he extended his life in the future.

*Dentures
Just Say No*

CHAPTER 15
Dentures – Just Say No

Removable teeth are at once a great help and a great difficulty for someone with missing teeth. For most, they're nothing more than oral wigs. They only mask a problem.

Unfortunately, bald gums aren't nearly as attractive as baldheads!

In essence, removable teeth are just devices that enable you to chew on your gums. The Bad News: the consequence of chewing on your gums is bone loss, loss of facial tone, more wrinkles and "old" looking faces.

Now for some, dentures have been successful. But for the majority of people, removable teeth are just a pain that changes the way their face looks, inhibits their ability to chew, and even causes facial disfigurement.

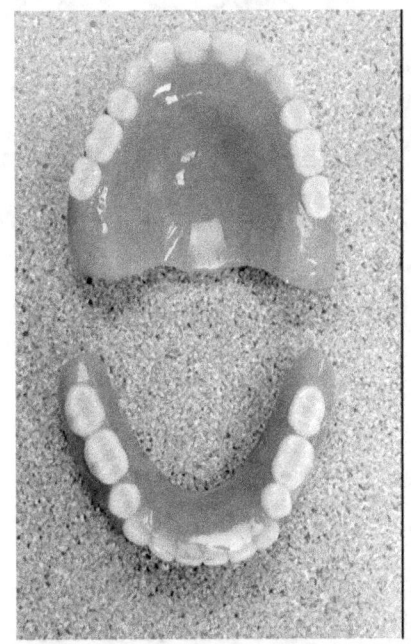

Upper and Lower Dentures

So if you're missing teeth, either don't get dentures, or if you must, get the best kind you possibly can.

Let's talk about the second option first. If you're going to wear dentures, understand that you have to be *kind* to your gums. It means you need to eat properly. You should take the nutritional supplements because your altered eating habits usually prevent chewing up the food you need for proper nutrition. If you're diabetic it's even <u>more important</u> that you keep your diabetes under control.

Why? Because the bone that supports those removable teeth melts away more quickly when your health is compromised, as with diabetes.

If you're going to have a denture or partial denture, make sure that they're done very well. Unfortunately removable dentures, whether a partial denture or full denture, are the place where people skimp the most. Some get the cheapest that they can.

And in 9 out of 10 cases the cheapest dentures cause them significant problems and money later on.

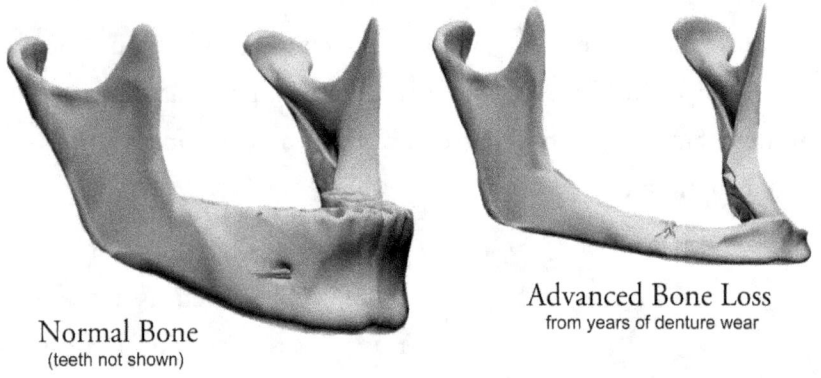

Normal Bone
(teeth not shown)

Advanced Bone Loss
from years of denture wear

Dentures do wear out. They have to be refitted. Unfortunately, the average denture wearer goes to the dentist every 14.9 years! This is wrong-headed thinking from lack of knowledge. Be Smart.

Within the first year of losing teeth, 60% of the width of bone in the upper jaw is lost. Gradually, over time, both the bone on the upper jaw and lower jaw begins to melt away. And as it melts away you have a decreasing ability to retain dentures. They move and feel insecure.

There are those that have musculature and tongue dynamics that allow them to wear dentures – very few. If <u>you</u> can manage removable teeth, that's great. Most people cannot.

But getting dental implants still would have been better than removable teeth.

For *some* people, removable teeth are the only solution, primarily because of economic realities. If you are to that point, try to have something called an overdenture.

An overdenture is a denture built over existing tooth roots. Tooth roots stimulate bone to remain. Tooth roots in the bone have nerve endings around them that give you a perception of bite force and give you orientation when you chew and eat. Overdentures allow you to chew with more force, more comfort, more ability, and help maintain the bone in your jaws.

Unfortunately, overdentures are frequently not implemented, or a patient's teeth are in such bad condition that overdentures aren't an option.

Speaking of upper and lower dentures, which denture do you think most people have trouble with? The lower. The upper can typically be made with a vacuum suction to stay in place and to have a good look.

The lower denture, on the other hand, is the usual culprit. You've got lots of muscle attachments in your lower jaw plus the tongue that tend to displace the lower denture. Furthermore, the loss of bone in the lower jaw compromises the ability for a lower denture to stay in place even more.

Remember this: your bite – how your teeth come together – is <u>critical</u> to long term denture success, as well as how much force you'll be able to use for every bite you take.

So, make sure that you find a good dentist who emphasizes getting a correct bite for your dentures. This can be difficult.

Making dentures is a process. Every one is different. Every individual person needs different things. And while you can get economy dentures, I suggest that if you're going to wear dentures, go with a premium version because more time, effort, care, skill and judgment will be used to create the premium dentures and that will help you look your best and chew most comfortably.

That being said, even the best dentist can have difficulty satisfying patients with dentures. **Anatomic realities simply make dentures difficult.**

On the other hand, you'd be amazed at the lengths that people go through to keep teeth that they shouldn't keep, just because they don't want to lose them. Never make the same mistake.

When you have diseased teeth that aren't going to get better, the longer you wait to take them out, the worse the infection gets, the more it affects your whole body.

Keeping bad teeth too long destroys bone levels and makes getting dental implants or even dentures far more difficult.

Dentures wear out. They have to be replaced. Thankfully, the number of people needing dentures has decreased dramatically. Fifty plus years of prevention has helped. Today more people have their teeth as they grow older.

So, what are the problems associated with removable teeth? **Over time your bite force decreases dramatically**. If you've been wearing dentures for 15 years or more, the amount of bite force can reduce to about 5 pounds per square inch. Your ability to eat and chew your food well goes out the window. Compare that to normal bite force of 25 - 250 lbs per square inch!

Denture wearers also face increased gastrointestinal disorders because they can't chew as well. Food poorly chewed takes its toll on your entire system. We believe you can <u>lose years</u> of life because of this inability to chew your food well.

Close to 90% of all patients with dentures claim some difficulty with speech. And 25% of people with dentures have very significant problems with them.

More than $200 million is spent each year on denture adhesives to help keep dentures in place and to avoid embarrassment. So, it's not just complete dentures that are a problem. Removable partial dentures are a problem, too.

The vast majority of denture wears using these adhesives need to have new dentures or refit their exsiting ones. Theses adhesives over-used can cause even more bone loss.

The survival rate of partial dentures is about 60% at four years. Which means that 40% of all removable partial dentures will be not used at four years. The survival rate of removable partial dentures at 10 years is only about 35%. This means that 6.5 out of 10 won't be used. Do you like these odds? I don't. You shouldn't either.

The teeth, to which the removable partial dentures attach themselves typically require far more repair. Over 60% of them, at six years, require some repair. After 10 years over 80% require some repair. Doesn't sound good to me. How about you?

Also, those teeth that help hold removable partial dentures in place suffer from increased movement. There's more plaque around them. The gum condition worsens and they're more likely to get decay.

Those who have removable partial dentures experience loss of teeth where removable partial dentures attach. A bit less than half of those teeth are lost within 10 years.

And there's also this problem: if one actually wears his removable partial denture, <u>accelerated</u> bone loss can come from chewing force.

These statistics are ugly.

It's estimated that those who wear partial dentures will often keep them in drawers because they feel uncomfortable wearing them and can actually chew better without them. Removeable teeth are second rate solutions.

Many people who wear complete dentures don't wear the lower one at all. It's not unusual for patients to have the upper one replaced and not have a lower denture at all.

If you have a choice between dentures and dental implants – go with dental implants. If you must have removeable dentures don't skimp. Get custom, personalized ones that distribute your bite force.

Unlike the slam-bam-thank-you-ma'am dentures that are made quickly and cheaply; premium dentures are the opposite. These multiple visits, precise impressioning, careful registration of the bite and careful selection of the best teeth for your best smile. Moreover, dentures like these can be made to give the best possible facial support. The result: dentures that help you look your best. Dentures that stay in place better. Dentures that are more stable and more comfortable. Many of our patients look so natural with these premium dentures that no one knows they are denture wearers! As you would imagine, dentures carefully engineered this way <u>are</u> more of an investment, and give much better results if you must wear dentures.

How do people end up losing all their teeth anyway?

Well, it doesn't occur because anyone plans on losing their teeth. Usually it is a result of ignorance, procrastination and false economy.

Too few people understand the consequences of choosing to lose a tooth and not replacing it.

Too few people realize the result of going years without having at least twice a year visits to a good dentist for maintaining their teeth.

Too many people put off the care they should have today until some uncertain time in the future. That future is always moving further and further away. Thinking "some day I'll get this done." That is the thinking that is a nice wish, but more a painful reality as dental problems start to snowball and more teeth are lost.

One tooth is lost, then another, and another. Then the answer seems to be "losing a tooth is the 'normal' way to treat dental problems." It isn't, unless a tooth is terminal.

For some people, the thinking becomes "I've already lost so many teeth, why not take this one out, too?" That is the sure road to tooth loss and future dental misery.

No one sets out to lose their teeth . Virtually everyone intuitively knows that keeping your teeth in a healthy condition provides an improvement in the quality of your life. Increasingly scientific evidence points to added years to a person's lifetime.

Procrastination Is Costly

Often people make bad choices because *at the time* expedient care seems to be a better decision. Unfortunately, removing teeth as a solution and not replacing them only delays problems - problems that get worse over time. Be warned. Get the best care you can as quickly as you can. Waiting years makes problems bigger, more difficult and far, far more expensive.

The Dilemma:

The older you are when you get dentures, the harder time you can have adapting to them. Everyone knows that your capacity to adapt physically decreases with age.

So you'd think that getting them at a younger age would be better because one has better adaptation abilities. While its true that you can adapt better when younger, it is also true the longer you wears dentures the more bone loss occurs.

You wouldn't imagine amputating a hand except under the direst of conditions, many treat teeth as nearly disposable!

As you grow older, your mouth typically gets drier. That's important because dentures "ride" on a thin layer of saliva. When you mouth gets dry, this saliva goes away and dentures cause increasingly worse problems - sore spots, pain and movement.

Reasons Why Dental Implants Are Preferred:

- Comfort
- Maintenance of the bone in your face.
- Maintenance of consistent jaw position in upper and lower. So when you bite together your face looks normal.
- Maintenance of the muscle tone in your face.
- Ability to speak more clearly.
- Able to chew more thoroughly, and get better nutrition.

All of these are good reasons to Say No to Dentures.

If you ask someone who has dentures and they are in a truthful mood, here is what they would say: "I'd rather have kept my teeth."

Jane's Story

"I didn't realize at the time what removing my teeth was going to do to me. I just wanted my pain to go away. I never liked dentists in particular anyway. I always associated visits with pain, anxiety and frankly, being expensive."

Jane had gushed out after I started our visit with a simple question: "Why are you here today?"

"I mean I was never clueless, what my choices were going to lead to," she continued.

"I resigned myself to the fact that I would just keep losing them and I would get dentures. But as I grow older and have heard the horror stories from my friends, I started to reconsider."

"Tell me about that," I inquired.

"Well, I thought that plates would be a good solution. Plus, the truth is I didn't want to spend the money to really get my teeth fixed. I mean there were so many other things that seemed more important at the time.

"Looking back now I realized what a huge mistake I made.

"It just seemed so much easier to take them out.

"Oh, money would have been tight, but what else is new!

"So here I am, doc. What can you do to help me?" she finished. Her face showed relief and acceptance from the dental confessional.

I knew what Jane needed. It wasn't a lecture on her dental sins of the past. She had been hard enough on herself already. No, she needed acceptance and hope.

"Jane, you've come to the right place. Those dark times of old-fashioned dentistry have come and gone. Let's not dwell on the past. It does no good. Yes, let's learn from it, and move forward. So you like that idea?" I offered.

She let out a sigh, smiled and said, "Thank you. I was so worried I was going to get a finger-wagging lecture. I had heard you were good with people like me. It looks like I've made the right choice."

She smiled at me and I smiled back.

We treated Jane with a set of premium dentures customized to her face, personality and jaw position.

After we had finished she told us how the new teeth were for her.

"I always get compliments on my smile now. I actually feel younger with my new teeth. No one realizes they are dentures."

It feels great to help people like Jane. These feelings of making a difference in someone else's life are what gives me professional satisfaction.

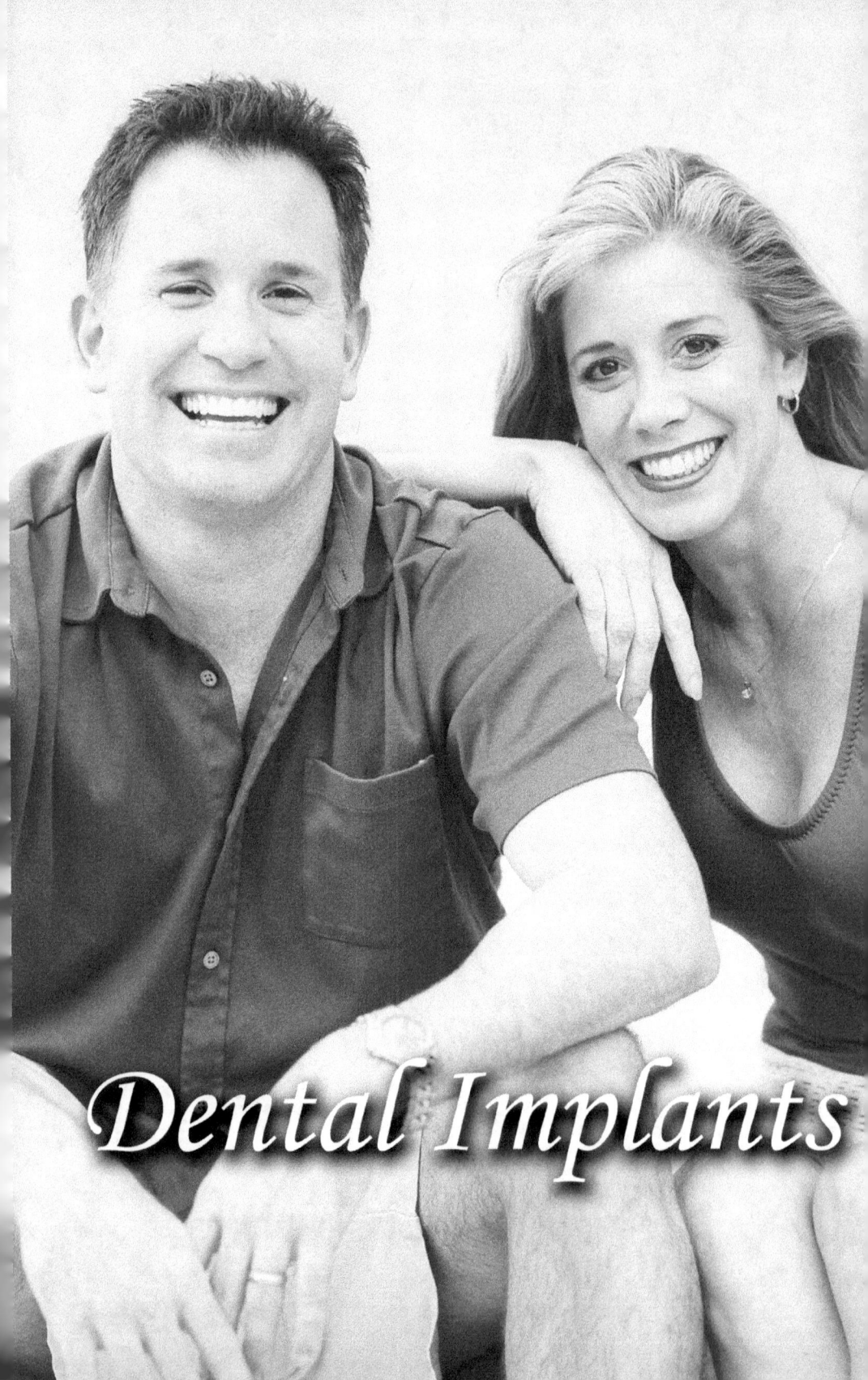

Dental Implants

CHAPTER 16
Dental Implants

"The mouth in its entirety is an important and even wondrous part of our anatomy, our emotions, and our life. It is the site of our very being. When an animal loses its teeth it cannot survive unless it's domesticated. Its very existence is terminated. It dies. In the human the mouth is the means of speaking, of expressing love, happiness and joy, anger, ill temper or sorrow. It is the primary sex contact; hence, it is of initial import to our regeneration and survival by food and propagation. It deserves the greatest care it can receive at any sacrifice."

- Dr. F. Harold Worth D.D.S.

What are dental implants? Dental implants are substitutes for tooth roots. That's a very simple definition, but one that's roughly true. Implants literally supply a third set of teeth for an individual who has lost a tooth or multiple teeth.

Implants can be different shapes, sizes and designs. But ultimately

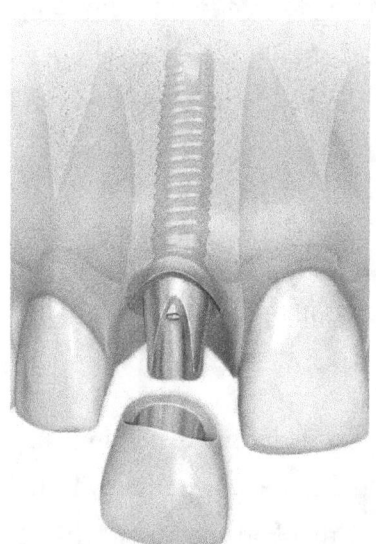

their purpose is to give fixed support using the bone of your jaws for replacement teeth.

How Are Implants Placed?

How are they placed? Generally an incision is made in the gum and the gum is pushed out of the way. A preparation of the bone is made and then an implant is seated into that preparation in the bone. The gum tissue is placed back and the bone around the implant heals around it, locking it into place. Then the implant can be used to anchor new teeth to the bone.

Then, depending upon the type of bone and the particular situation, the implant is either allowed to heal for a number of months or put into use right away. The speed of putting the implant into use varies depending on a number of factors including location, type and volume of bone, chewing function and other factors. A typical time frame is four to six months after surgical placement.

Kimberly's Story

Let me tell you a little story about Kimberly. Kimberly had a hard time as a child and teenager. Through her own drive and determination she managed to overcome her difficulties, including a broken family, lack of money and education.

When Kimberly came to me her mouth was, as so many patients say, a "dental disaster". She proclaimed, "I know I'm a train wreck."

Kimberly had a good deal of dentistry done, a lot of it not done very well. She had chosen the most economical choices, although not the best choices for her. And she had a lot of what we call Scotch-Tape dentistry.

She was then in a position where she could no longer afford her prior level of care because she had already lost over half her teeth and the others were on the way downhill. They were sure to go if she continued as she was.

So, we did a number of things for her including dental implants to replace those missing teeth. Today Kimberly is smiling. She has a family and an executive position with a Fortune 500 firm.

She comes in regularly to have her maintenance therapy and checkups. Kimberly is just one of millions of people who have availed themselves of dental implants.

Dramatic Increase in the Use of Dental Implants

So, why has the use of dental implants increased so dramatically? Why have dental implants become the solution for the replacement of missing teeth?

They are a preferred solution for a number of reasons. One reason is that with implants, you isolate all your therapy on just the area where the missing tooth or teeth were so other teeth don't have to be touched. Number two is they have excellent success and impressive longevity; typically 90% of implants last 15 to 20 years or more.

And implants are comfortable. Often a patient will say, "Well, I don't want to have this done because I'm afraid of the pain associated with it." This is understandable because of the prior history a patient may have had with dental therapy many years ago. But, that was back in the old-fashioned days when dentistry

> ### What Is a Dental Implant?
>
> A dental implant is a biocompatible man-made substitute that replaces missing tooth roots. It's usually made of a space age alloy of titanium and comes in various shapes and sizes. Most are cylinders placed into bone and left undisturbed while the bone heals around them, locking them in like an anchor.
>
> After a few months the implants are used as a foundation for replacing the missing teeth. Dental implants restore lost chewing ability, improve appearance and relieve embarrassment and give real self-confidence to patients who need them. For many, they really are a true breakthrough.

could be quite difficult. No more. Today, once we finish placing the implant, the typical patient statement is, "Wow, that was far easier than I expected. And to think how I worried about it. That was one of the easiest things I have ever had done!"

Tim's Story

A patient named Tim came to us with just a single missing tooth. He wanted to do something about it, but didn't want to cut down his adjacent teeth.

So, for Tim, it was a pretty simple procedure. We placed his implant and because of his bone density and his particular circumstances, we were able to put an artificial tooth on right away. It wasn't a final one, but it was a provisional one that allowed him to get rid of that space almost immediately.

After a number of months we put the final crown in place. Now Tim smiles very proudly.

Implants are certainly easier than many other types of mouth surgeries. And they also have the distinct advantage of not being susceptible to decay. You can't get a cavity in an implant.

Implants are made of biocompatible materials, typically some alloy of titanium. These alloys are light and strong and the body seems to adore them. The bone heals around the implant and locks it into place.

The Missing Side View Tooth

It's common for those with a single missing tooth on the side to think it doesn't show when they smile. Does it show from the front? Maybe not. But it almost always shows from the side. And that can look very degrading, unfortunately. A dental implant can make a huge difference here.

Should A Diseased Tooth Be Repaired Or Should It Be Removed And Have An Implant Placed?

More and more these days, we are removing very diseased teeth and placing dental implants as the solution. This requires a good dentist who can help you make the right choice.

Implants will help to preserve the bone and the jaw. They preserve the bite position, which will shift if missing teeth are allowed to continue to be missing.

And by the way, missing teeth in one arch, upper or lower jaw, have a direct effect on the teeth in the opposing

> **The indications for dental implant therapy:**
>
> A. When you have lost a single tooth.
>
> B. When you have already lost several teeth.
>
> C. When a whole side of teeth are gone.
>
> D. When an entire jaw of teeth are gone, upper or lower.
>
> E. When you need a complete upper and lower replacement of all teeth.

arch. This means, for example, that if you have missing teeth on the lower left, the teeth on the upper left will be affected, because those upper teeth will erupt towards the empty spots.

And when they do, you put healthy teeth at risk of becoming unhealthy. As they change positions, food begins to get trapped, plaque has its way and gum disease ensues. Moreover, these otherwise healthy teeth move into the space that should be occupied by the lower teeth. This alone can cause the loss of the upper teeth. It's not a pretty picture.

Thus, implants also have the benefit of helping you *maintain your existing teeth*.

Are there risks associated with dental implants? Yes, there are, but these are relatively low. Not all implants work. Of course, nothing works all the time. If you have missing teeth or a missing tooth, you had natural teeth that didn't work.

But the good news is, with today's technology, success rates are over 90% at 10 years plus. And in some cases 95+% over 20 years. That is a higher success rate than conventional dentistry!

Amongst all types of implants placed in the body, dental implants are the most successful.

What are the implications of not having missing teeth replaced?

It's the accelerated effect dental problems have on your face, on how much you age, and on your ability to consume food. Why? Because obviously if you can't chew as well, you won't be able to consume food as well.

And what of nutrition? If you have to change your diet because of your teeth, it can't help but affect your health. Let me explain why.

If your ability to chew well suffers, you have to change to softer foods. And what's characteristic of those softer foods? Higher carbohydrate content, literally more starches and more sugars. This increased carbohydrate intake can lead to obesity and diabetes.

Obesity is a major problem in this country, affecting virtually 60% of the adult population of America. It's one of the reasons you see the ubiquity of diet and weight control ads throughout the television and the Internet.

With this change in nutrition comes a change in your health. What goes in has a direct effect on your body's ability to function.

Also, as you probably realize, with obesity comes an increased risk of pre-diabetes and actual diabetes, the chronic scourges of the body that tear it down and make for unpleasant living, chronic disease and cardiovascular problems. Sadly, the pre-diabetic doesn't understand his risk. There are 57 million pre-diabetics, millions will become diabetic.

How Long Do Dental Implants Take?

How long do dental implants take to complete? The time can vary from a few months to a couple of years, when bone and tissue must be re-built first. The time needed is dependent upon an individual's situation. For some, it's relatively quick – a few months. They can have teeth removed at one appointment and implants placed at the same time and walk out having teeth in place. These won't be final teeth, but there will be teeth in place. Most frequently, implant placement and restoration takes 5 to 8 months.

How Long Do Implants Last?

Dentists are now seeing some implants that have lasted 30 years and more. Several things have to be done for implants to be successful. First, they have to be properly diagnosed.

The second thing is that they have to be properly placed. And they have to be placed in such a way that your body will accept them. Implants must be bioengineered so that bite forces are spread out properly to the bone. Too few implants will not pass these forces on properly.

Third, they have to be taken care of. People who failed to take care of their original teeth could have trouble if the implants are not cared for well. You can get peri-implant disease, literally meaning disease around the implant, as a result of poor home care. Is it a big problem? No, but it can be.

How can you help? Understand what implants are, not to expect more than they can accomplish, or for that matter, too little.

Implants can be a major miracle for a whole number of people to help them maintain their smile and chew properly while protecting any adjacent teeth from excessive stress.

Mistakes with Dental implants

What are some mistakes that people make with dental implants?

- **Too Few Implants to Replace Missing Teeth**

Often patients come to me for second opinions about dental implants. The most frequent situation is a patient or inexperienced doctor wanting to place too few implants to take the load of the bite and chewing.

Understand this: an implant is "like" a tooth root, a little better in some ways, a little worse in others. How is it better? Well, it does not get decay. It's less likely to get gum disease than natural teeth. How is it not as good? It can't take sideways force as well. Your teeth are built with little microscopic sized ligaments around them that allow some "give" when force is applied to them. These little ligaments are called periodontal ligaments. These allow some side forces to be withstood quite well.

Dental implants work best with forces in an up and down direction on them, what we call compressive force. They do quite well with that.

Dealing with Stress

Too much stress can cause the loss of an implant, as well as a tooth.

What is the stress I am speaking of here? It is not the stress of daily living. It is the stress of biomechanical force.

The definition of stress in dentistry is how much force is distributed over how wide an area. An easy way to think about this: snowshoes. When walking in deep snow, a regular shoe plunges down into the snow. There is too much force concentrated on too small an area. Snowshoes distribute your weight (force) over a wide area allowing you to walk on top of the snow. The larger the area engaged for support, the greater the distribution of force and the less the stress. Managing the biomechanical forces of function is a key part of successful implant therapy.

Can you imagine what the problem of too few implants? Too little area to distribute the force. The implants lose bony support due to excessive stress placed on them and the supporting bone.

The same can be true if you were missing a bunch of teeth on one side of your mouth. You have to put all your chewing force on the remaining teeth. When there are too few teeth, there's too much force. And with too much force, the teeth get loose. So whether teeth or implants are involved, too much force on too few teeth causes them to lose bone and fail over time.

Too few implants are a major mistake that's made when placing implants.

How Many Implants Should be Used?

A general rule of thumb is that if you're missing one tooth, you need one implant. The exception to that rule is with molar implants. Because these are the largest teeth in the mouth and were designed to bear the brunt of chewing force, often two implants are need for a single missing molar.

If you're missing two smaller teeth, you need two implants. If you're missing three teeth, it's often three implants. If you're missing four teeth, often it's only three implants. If you're missing five teeth it's going to be somewhere between three and four implants. If you're missing six teeth it's generally somewhere between three and four implants. If you're missing a whole arch of teeth it's going to range from, depending on the individual, from five to nine implants. This is determined based on the person's size, ability to bring force and what is being chewed against in the opposite jaw. Chewing against natural teeth or other implants requires more implants for support because they are so much better at highly efficient chewing forces.

The number of implants that are used to replace missing teeth is customized to each patient, dependent upon an individual's situation.

All of dentistry is customized. It's based upon individual diagnosis and what needs to be done. Back to our mistakes with dental implants:

- **Too Little Treatment to Fully Solve the Problems:**

Akin to the problem of too few implants is skimping on care, doing too little to actually solve the problem.

Please don't make this mistake.

I've had patients before who said, "Well, I want to get this done with few implants and build all these replacement teeth on top of them for X dollars."

This is the classic example of doing too little. Doing too little is a waste of money. It would be like paying to fly a jet across the country and only paying for fuel to get you one third of the way. You are going to crash. Similarly, too little treatment to "do it right" is asking for it all to crash and burn.

I recommend that nothing be done in these skimping situations. It would be better to spend your time and money on something you can enjoy than to waste your time and money on an incomplete care that has a poor chance of success.

Of course, there can be alternatives to implants to reduce the investment in care. While there may be only one diagnosis, there can be many ways to treat. If you must spend less than needed to get a complete implant job done, use an alternative plan that does complete the work, albeit quite differently.

Obviously, no one would dream of trying to build a house without a firm foundation or a strong roof. Without a foundation, the house will wash away. Without a roof it can't be protected. Trying to skimp on your dental care is a lot like that. It's like not having a foundation or not having a good roof.

You should have this understanding: dental implantology is the most challenging of all facets of dentistry. While it is not a specialty in and of itself, it requires virtually every other discipline of dentistry to perform very well. It requires understanding of bioengineering, biomechanics, biofunctionality, biology of the teeth and bone, bone density, bone shape, contour position. It requires understanding of physics and force vectors. It requires an understanding of precise surgical techniques and human anatomy. It requires an understanding and application of all parts of dentistry to perform very well.

Because of these complexities with dental implants, fees are often substantially higher than everyday dentistry.

- **Failing to Find Out Why You Had Trouble in the Past**

Why have you lost your teeth? That answer becomes important for your future.

Do the reasons that you originally lost your teeth still exist? If they do, can they be removed? How likely is it that those problems could come back again? These are important questions because the answers help determine the probabilities of more teeth being lost. Has the situation stabilized so it is unlikely to happen again? What are the potential future problems? How likely are they to occur?

This is where a good dentist will do "The Humphrey Bogart." In the famous classic movie, Casablanca, Humphrey Bogart must make a decision for himself and the love of his life, Ingrid Bergman. He had to decide what was best for everyone, in spite of his own feelings and life. This is what we are often faced with in complex care like dental implants. A good dentist will think for the both of you. What is best based on what we now know? The treatment can be a huge investment. A good dentist will plan your care so the least amount of work possible is dependent on all the other parts. This segmental approach means that if one particular facet of the dental work fails for whatever reason, then all the other work can be saved and remain useful and working. This gives a far simpler fix, easier care, increased longevity of treatment, and can save you thousands of dollars

- **An Inexperienced or Poorly Trained Dentist**

A mistake too, is not having someone who fully understands dental implants and all of its facets. You need an experienced, well-trained dentist for dental implants. Dental implants take special training; make sure your dentist has it.

- **Failing to Do Your Part**

Another mistake that's made is failing to do your part with your home care and following instructions. You have to partner with your dentist on this. If you fail to do your part, you could doom any work, no matter how good the dentist is.

Good home care takes a little bit of time to get use to. It will take more than thirty seconds of tooth brushing with a dab of tooth-paste to take good care of your new smile. We often find that many patients still do not know everything they should about caring for their teeth and gums!

The good news is that we will teach you this. We'll show you how to care for your mouth so it can stay healthy. When you know how, it gets a whole lot easier and often faster. The hassle can virtually disappear!

You will have to get used to the idea it's going to take some time. If you're not willing to spend some time taking care of your teeth, don't expect them to last and don't expect your implants to last either.

You have the responsibility to follow the dentist's instructions on home care and the use of your teeth including foods to eat and not eat(especially during healing times.)

• Not Knowing Enough to Choose Wisely

Another mistake is in not knowing enough to choose wisely. Dental implants can be a significant investment. And I say significant investment I mean from thousands or tens of thousands of dollars. And those tens of thousands can extend to a six figure range in severe situations.

Understand this: the more you need done and the more you want your teeth to look like, feel like, and function like natural teeth, the greater the fee will be.

Trying to cut corners inevitably gets you in trouble. A concept I've mentioned before is over-engineering. Over-engineering is your ticket to making sure that the metals and restorative materials that are used do not get over stressed as a result of functional use. This means they have the capacity to last for decades.

You had the insight to be reading this book, so you will know how to choose wisely.

• Incomplete Diagnosis and Workup

Another mistake is not having a complete workup and diagnosis. Doing a complete workup and diagnosis where warranted, takes significant time and dollars.   It takes multiple kinds of x-rays, often oral photography, molds and impressions of your existing teeth, lab work. The list gets longer as your problems increase. Making the time and effort to get this done is your best assurance against incomplete or under-diagnosed care.

How could you get the best care possible without getting a complete diagnosis? How can you know and understand your problems without a full work-up? Your diagnostic work-up should be customized specifically to you as an individual.

- **"Well, I'll just accept what I've got."**

Another mistake is just kind of brushing all this off and saying, "Well, I'll just accept what I've got." Unfortunately that laissez-faire approach to your teeth may be what got you in trouble with your teeth in the first place.

Choosing to ignore your teeth is a near certain road to mouth problems. Moreover, once your problems start, they inevitably multiply.

The more trouble you have with your teeth, the more active you have to be in caring for them. You should be proactive rather than waiting on something else bad to happen.

It is important for you to **do something about your situation**.

On the other side, don't let over analysis cause paralysis. This can occur quite easily when you go through too many choices. Narrow your choices down and choose the dentist you can trust based on experience, training, talent, results and relationship.

The wonderful thing about the Internet is there's a lot of information to be found. The disappointment about the Internet is you can easily get partial truths or outright false information. Both can be very detrimental. While what is said on the internet can be accurate, a particular piece of information may not apply to you or just be wrong. While you need information; you also **need to have a trusted advisor to guide you, a dentist who "knows the business" about dental implants**.

- **Living on that Island called "Someday I'll"**

Another mistake is living on that island called "Someday I'll". It never comes. I encourage you, if you have missing teeth, to go ahead and get something done about it. Procrastination is deadly when it comes to dental care.

Find a capable practitioner who can help you.

So, just skip "Someday I'll" and go straight to the land of "I Did It and Now I'm Smiling."

- **"I was told I couldn't have dental implants."**

From time to time a new patient will tell us what another dentist has told them:

"I was told I couldn't have dental implants"

> or

"Another dentist said I didn't have enough bone"

> or

"I wasn't a good candidate."

While all of these statements *may be* true, the real truth could be that the dentist doesn't like using dental implants. The dentist may not be trained in the use of implants. The dentist may not recognize what is possible. This is happening less these days as more dentists are becoming knowledgeable about the use of dental implants.

Sometimes patients don't have enough bone to place an implant. That does not preclude, or prevent you from having implants placed. What do I mean? Usually we're able to graft bone, stimulate bone growth or transplant bone from one part of the jaw to the next to have enough bone for implant placement.

Unfortunately, the "you're not a good candidate" remark often comes from those who are untrained and don't understand dental implants. Is it sometimes true that you aren't a good candidate? Yes, it is sometimes true, but close to 95% of all patients typically are good candidates!

If you have significant health factors, you smoke two packs of cigarettes a day and have very poor home care or if you're an uncontrolled diabetic, then I'd say you're <u>not</u> a good candidate.

Speaking of that, what about someone who has diabetes, can they have dental implants? The answer is yes. We do that frequently. The person with diabetes needs to be under good control and stay under control for long-term success.

Different Kinds of Implant Replacement Teeth

There are different kinds of replacement teeth that can be built on dental implants. First is what we call fixed in place teeth. **Fixed in place** means that once the teeth go into place, they do not come out. Teeth placed this way are usually cemented into place or sometimes placed with screws. This is the way most people prefer using dental implants because it is most like having one's natural teeth.

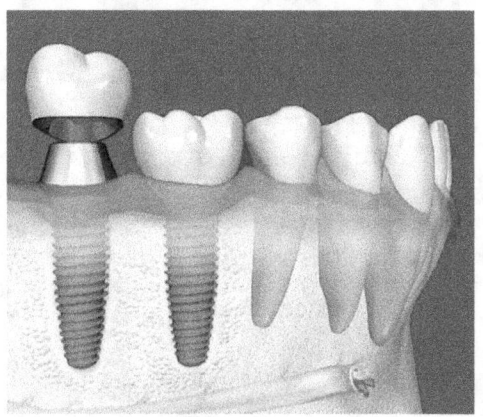

This method has the added advantage of the longevity of the replacement teeth themselves. Unlike the other two methods explained here late, this type of restoration does not have to be redone or replaced as often because they last longer.

The second type of implant restoration is what we call **semi-fixed teeth**. Semi-fixed teeth are quite stable, function well as teeth and are removable. Because these are removable, these generally have more parts that move. More moving parts mean more potential for wear or other trouble.

Semi-fixed teeth clip or snap into place. This is used when entire arches need replacing. Therefore, this is not a usable method when just a single tooth or a section of teeth are being replaced.

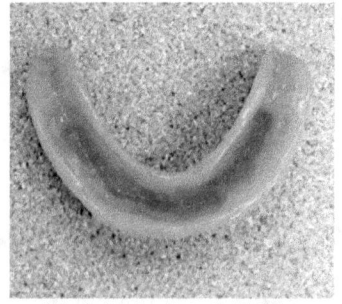

Clip in Teeth: Note Gold Clips

For a few people, this is their preferred restoration as it gives them more access to clean the implants under the replacement teeth. However, most patients find the fixed in place teeth a better choice.

Because these teeth are removable, they use clips, snaps, or o-rings to anchor the replacement teeth. Unfortunately, these, too, wear out and require replacing. The frequency of attachment replacement is from three to twenty-four months.

Semi-fixed teeth have the advantage of typically costing less than fixed in place, and the disadvantage of having to be replaced after a number of years, typically because of the wear of the replacement teeth.

How often the semi-fixed teeth need replacing due to wearing out varies. The implants may be perfectly fine, but the teeth that are supported by the implants will wear out with semi-fixed. I have had patients who need replacing every three years and others that last fifteen. It is an individual rate depending on the use of the teeth. If the patient clenches or grinds his teeth, the teeth fail faster. The heavier the function and use, the faster the replacement required. An average lifespan for replacement of semi-fixed teeth on implants is seven years.

The third method is also the third choice in preference. Removable teeth with implant retention uses fewer implants, often just two, to help hold a denture in place. This has the advantage of lesser costs, but the enormous disadvantage of continuing loss of bone over time. The removable teeth move around more and give up the advantages of the first two methods in preserving bone.

Removable teeth with implant retention helps prevent the removable denture from moving around a lot. The dental implants give the denture some stability so it moves less. For some people this can be a real aid. This is the least suggested treatment because it fails to preserve bone like the other two methods. In fact, the increased chewing ability afforded by this method can hasten the demise of bone because of the increased compressive force on the unprotected bone.

What's New in Dental Implants?

So, what's new in dental implants? What's possible now that didn't used to be?

How Can Implants Improve Your Looks?

Dental implants can improve your looks by helping to provide bone support, replacing missing teeth and preserving the bony structures of the face. Those bony structures are the support for your facial muscles and skin. You need them. No amount of make up or face lift can replace that critical bone. A sure fire way to look older is to lose that critical bone. Without the teeth, you can become a dental cripple, condemned to the foods you can mush around or suck through a straw.

For many people, dental implants can be a modern miracle that changes not only how they look, but also how they feel about their life. They can help you have a big broad smile that will make other less pleasing parts of your face less important, what we call the smile dominant face. This is such a boon to the older person. The wrinkles one invariably gets with age seemingly melt away when you flash that big, broad, beautiful smile that's possible with dental implants.

Today we have different sizes, lengths and types of implants that allow us to do implants in places we couldn't before.

We're now able to grow bone to replace missing bone using bone grafts, bone growth factors and new bone gaining surgical techniques so that implants can be placed like never before.

We are also now combining other facets of dentistry with dental implants to improve appearances, to improve functionality and put smiles on people's faces all the time.

Dental implants are even being used in orthodontic treatment and orthognathic surgery. Orthognathic surgery is the surgery of the upper and/or lower jaw to change the shape of the face and improve the bite position. It is frequently used in adult ortho-dontics, problems of growth in children and teenagers, and facial trauma. Implants used this way are being used as anchors for tooth movement and bone stability.

How Happy are People With Dental Implants?

So, here's a question. How happy are people who've had implants done? That's an important question. I would say that a fair assessment is somewhere around 98% of people would say, "If I had to choose again, I would do it again."

When you ask about comfort, they would say, "I was surprisingly comfortable throughout the whole procedure."

When asked, "Knowing what you know now, would you recommend dental implants to other people?" And the answer's almost invariably "yes."

Should you Gamble with Your Years?

Trying to time your healthcare, based on how long you're going to live is just not a good idea. It may seem appealing on the one hand because you think, "I won't spend this money". But on the other hand if a family member or a loved one knew that you were doing that they would probably not like it and probably would want you to do everything you could to help stay healthy.

So, what should you do? Number one, if you have missing teeth, get them replaced, preferably with dental implants if you're a good candidate for them.

How Much Do Dental Implants Cost?

This is one of the main questions that come across on the Internet searches, how much do implants cost?

Fees can range a lot. A single implant placement (without the replacement teeth), on the low side can be $1,500 to the high side of $4,000. Part of that depends upon your location, the care, skill and judgment of the practitioner providing them and the cost and materials they use.

An implant itself is only part of the fee though, and this should be understood. Because in addition to placing the implant, there also has to be surgery associated with uncovering it. Placing the replacement teeth onto the implants is often times a significantly larger part of the total fees than just placing the implant itself.

When multiple implants are needed, fees grow accordingly. The more you want the replacement teeth to look and function like natural teeth, the higher the fees can go. The good news is that 98% of patients having implants done say it was worth the fee.(As for the other 2%, the majority were happy with their care, they just didn't like paying that much for it.)

Can you be too young or too old to get implants?

That's a good question. Let's take the young one first. Generally speaking good dentists want individuals to have stopped growing, their jaws to have stopped growing before implants are place.

For young girls, age 15 is typically the age that they stop having changes in the bone plates.

With young men, typically that age is somewhere between 18 and 21. Again, we typically want to wait until all growth is completed before implants are placed.

Frequently implants are used to replace congenitally missing teeth and this can be a real panacea for those who have that problem.

How to Choose an Implant Dentist

How do you find a good implant dentist? How do you find one who does dental implants on a regular basis and has the requisite experience with them?

Ask the dentist about his training and experience with dental implants. Ask him or her to show you before and after pictures of cases done.

Be wary of anyone who treats dental implants as a minor part of care. Dental implants are a major part of care and need to have that type of importance attached to them.

Understand that a practitioner who does them all the time, will sometimes fail to explain things as much as someone who doesn't. Why? Because they're so used to placing implants that they may assume you understand and may not explain things as well as they should. Keep asking until you understand.

But we need to wait until they finish growing to do that.

How about too old? Well, there really isn't a too old factor. And this is a very interesting question. Age alone is not a determining factor.

I've had patients in their late 80's, early 90's say yes to treatment with dental implants and been quite successful.

In fact, one patient, I can't reveal his entire name but we'll call him John, (a kind man who had one of the deepest voices I've ever heard in my life) told me that as a result of his dental implants he feels like it saved his life.

I asked why he felt that way and he said, "Well, I was so sick." He had cancer treatment. "I was so sick before, if I hadn't had these teeth where I could actually eat again, I don't think I would have made it." So, John's still with us, thank God.

Again, age alone is not a determining factor. Some people like to play the guessing game of "how long am I going to live". Understand this, we're all living longer, we're going to need our teeth longer. And over 50% of those people that are age 60 right now or will be, are going to live into their 90's or even 100's. So why choose implants if you are older?

For some it's about living a longer life. And for others it's about preserving their health for a lifetime. And for others it's just simply, "I want my teeth to look good and feel good. And not to be another worry for me, in other words, I want piece of mind."

All of these are great reasons to have dental implants.

We have the social pleasure of dining and dating and being with other people throughout our entire life. For many people, dental implants help maintain that social pleasure, whether they're traveling, meeting someone new or just working on a job.

As you can see, dental implants have many, many benefits. It's a shame when people don't avail themselves of that advantage.

Who benefits from having implant dentistry?

1. Denture wearers who are frustrated and tired of the problems with full dentures and partial dentures. These problems can consist of:

    □ the 'goo' that they use to keep them in place

    □ the pain they associate with biting and chewing

□ the embarrassment of teeth that can literally fly out on their plate. This is kind of what we call Murphy's Law of denture movement, it happens at the worst possible time.

2. Those who have bone loss that is literally causing the lack of support for their face or causing ugly disfiguring appearances to the face, including extra wrinkling and lines.

3. Those who have missing teeth or who are about to lose teeth due to decay or fracture.

4. Accident victims from motor vehicle accidents, football or other sports injuries.

5. Those that have a mouth full of problems that just seem to get worse and worse.

6. Those who have otherwise perfect teeth except for one or two missing teeth.

7. Those who are committed to a high level of dental health will benefit from implant dentistry.

Dental implants can be a real miracle for those who have been frustrated with earlier attempts to fix their teeth, those who want to recapture their youthful appearance, those who've had significant gum disease. And it's for those people who feel they are dental disasters with no place to turn.

Should You Have Dental Implants?

The number of implants used in the United States has grown significantly over the past years. Back in 1983 very little was done with dental implants, only about $10 million was spent for dental implants by dentists. (That isn't what the public spent.)

Dental Implants
Here's How It Works

The steps of the implant procedure itself: If there is a damaged tooth that must be removed, it is removed comfortably. Once the tooth is removed an assessment is made on whether to place an implant at the same time or let the site heal where the tooth was.

If the site needs to heal, a bone graft is placed to help preserve bone while it's healing. Once the bone is healed, a small implant is placed in that space. You can think of the implant like a grooved or threaded titanium post.

Your body begins to bond to this titanium post right away. It can take somewhere between three and six months before we can go to the next step.

Your body does not reject these materials but ties in with them with great strength, as if they were a natural part of your body.

Once a titanium implant is tightly in place a post, like a dowel is now attached down into and on top of the dental implant. Often these are screwed into place.

And then a new tooth is made to fit on top of this post. Voila! You have a new tooth and you're the only one who knows it's manmade.

In fact, implants are so comfortable you'll soon forget what one is. Your body thinks it's your own and so will you.

Today hundreds of millions of dollars are spent in placing and helping patients with dental implants. Why are implants and the implant related treatments on the rise?

We have an aging population that's living longer. And as people live longer, people lose more teeth. So, there's more of a need for them.

For some people there's old dentistry that has worn out and teeth that have failed and they have to be replaced using dental implants. There's the problem that people have with wearing dentures and removable partial dentures. Frankly dentures are poor substitutes for natural teeth but the best we had before dental implants.

Of course, there are consequences of wearing removable dentures, which include loss of bone in the jaws, increased wrinkling, and loss of bite function. There are also the psychological losses associated with tooth loss and the feeling of not being whole.

And for many baby boomers this is something they absolutely reject. They want to feel whole. They want to feel complete. They want to feel that they have lived a full, complete life.

As the population tends to grow older they want to live active lives. And they do not want to be put on the shelf.

A second reason for the increased use of implants is the predictable long-term results of implant supported replacement teeth. And, of course, then there are the advantages of implant-supported teeth; their durability, their appearance, their functionality. All of those are reasons for having dental implants.

One of the big reasons, that I encourage patients to have dental implants, particularly those who are working to avoid removable teeth or are trying to get out of removable teeth, is the effect it has on their nutrition and their total health.

You don't really want to be in a nursing home where you're going to get unpredictable care by low paid workers who either don't care or don't understand your particular needs related to your teeth. And it's not uncommon for people in nursing homes to have their dentures lost and never found again or have dentures returned to them that don't even belong to them.

So, for some, dental implants can be the right answer for preventing nutritional problems. This alone is often enough to prevent going into a nursing home and living out your last years in those places, warehoused and drugged into compliant behavior.

So, for the 70 year-old patient who is debating whether to spend tens of thousands of dollars on having dental implants placed, the question is "Is it worth it at my age?" And the answer is yes, because they could have up to two decades or more of their life to live.

Adapting to removable teeth can be a really uncomfortable experience for someone who's in their 70's and 80's or 90's.

So, what are some other benefits of dental implants? They can dramatically reduce or even eliminate your emotional anguish about your current smile. And they can actually improve your health and longevity. Dental implants often help one to stop sacrificing foods that you love for the ones that your dentures and missing teeth allow you to have.

So, what can dental implants do for you? They can rejuvenate; literally dazzle your smile again. They can make you feel whole again. Help you regain lost function. They can help you, get noticed by that special someone that you want noticing you.

For some it's saving your health. For others it gives them back a youthful vibrancy they've lost many years ago. For some, it lets them look 10 to 20 years younger.

For others, it's avoiding the embarrassment of loose dentures or missing teeth, making for awkward social situations that no one wants. It'll enable you to eat the foods you want, to chew comfortably and with confidence. And for some, it's rekindling romance that was lost.

Are You a Candidate for Dental Implants?

Still not sure if you're a good candidate for dental implants? Here's a quiz to find out. Check all that apply to you.

_____ Pain on chewing.

_____ Anxiety about your smile.

_____ Difficulty in dealing with stress.

_____ Unattractive smile.

_____ Social embarrassment.

_____ Difficulty in sleeping.

_____ Difficulty in swallowing.

_____ You had to have a change in the foods you eat.

_____ Shrinking bone.

_____ Must use denture adhesives.

_____ A gag reflex.

_____ A need to feel whole again.

_____ Bad breath that won't go away.

_____ Difficulty in relationships because of your teeth.

_____ Feel older than you are.

_____ Loss of self esteem.

_____ Depression over your teeth.

_____ Difficulty in chewing.

_____ Mouth sores.

_____ Difficulty in speaking.

_____ Unstable teeth.

_____ Unstable dentures.

_____ Burning sensations without your own teeth.

_____ Numbness in the face and lips.

_____ Headaches.

_____ Withdrawals from social interaction or events.

_____ Food trapped between or under your teeth.

_____ Food trapped between or underneath your replacement dentures.

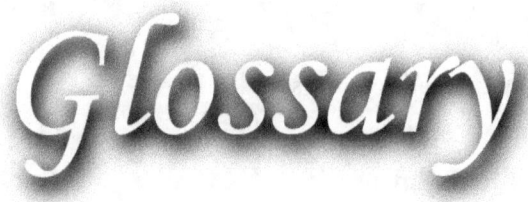

A1C level The volume of glycated hemoglobin in your blood, used to measure the long-term average of blood glucose. Glycated red blood cells cause microvascular damage that can result in blindness, kidney disease, nerve damage, heart attack and stroke.

Alveolar bone The socket that your tooth sits in. It's actually two bones – one is the socket itself and the other is a structural support, sort of like the joists that sit on beams to provide support for the floor in your house. This structure provides a firm anchor point for your tooth.

C-reactive protein (CRP) When the body senses inflammation somewhere in the system, it signals the liver to produce CRP. As inflammation worsens, the level of CRP in your blood rises. CRP is associated with both diabetes and gum disease, and is a predictor of heart disease and stroke.

Gingivitis A mild form of gum disease. You may hear dental health professionals refer to the 'gingiva'. That's the clinical term for your gums. Gingivitis often develops when plaque builds up on your teeth at the gumline and irritates the gum.

Inflammation response Sensing irritation, the body responds with an automatic system that's a defense mechanism against inflammation. This is a complex set of events that send several different types of cells to the site. These cells have specific jobs that are designed to remove whatever is causing the irritation and help the tissue that's been injured to start to heal.

Macrovascular Pertaining to the body's major arteries and veins. These are the sites for arterial plaques and blood clots which can cause heart attack or stroke.

Microvascular Involving the smallest structures of the circulatory system, including venules, capillaries and arterioles. These connect with progressively smaller pathways, ultimately delivering nutrients to individual cells. In these sites, damage can be done to the eyes, kidneys, and lower extremities, areas that are particularly vulnerable to effects of diabetes.

Periodontal ligaments Connective tissues that do just that – they connect the cementum and the gum to the alveolar bone.

Periodontitis Put in its most simple terms, periodontitis is gum disease. The literal meaning of the word 'periodontal' is straightforward – 'peri' means 'around', and 'dont' means 'tooth'. So, periodontal refers to the parts of your mouth that surround your tooth. The word 'periodontitis' refers to the diseases that affect these parts of your mouth. These are generally bacterial infections that attack the gums and other oral components. See Chapter Two for types of periodontal diseases.

Phagocytes Cells that can engulf and kill other cells, such as the bacteria that are attacking your gums in periodontal disease. With your normal defenses lowered by diabetes, the bacteria can enter the bloodstream and trigger the body's inflammation response as well as attack major organs such as the heart and kidneys.

Porphyromonous gingivalis One of the most common pathogens in periodontal disease. If you have periodontal disease the risk of being infected with this pathogen is more than 11 times greater. This bacteria enters the bloodstream and travels throughout the body, and is believed to play a role in developing coronary artery disease that can lead to heart attack or stroke.

Meet Dr. Marcius

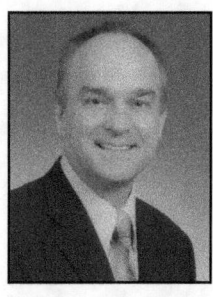

Dr. Marcius is a general dentist who provides cosmetic dentistry, dental implants and IV sedation. After more than 25 years in practice and advanced training in cosmetic dentistry, implant dentistry and jaw joint dysfunction, he has acquired the tools to solve some of dentistry's most complex cases. He treats patients experiencing a wide-range of dental problems, from routine cleanings to total mouth reconstructions. Using his artistic skill-set acquired from experience with paint and photography, Dr. Marcius continues to design beautiful, natural smiles his patients love.

Training

- University of Akron (Biology, Chemistry)
- Case Western Reserve University

Post Doctoral Training

- Miami Valley Hospital/Sinclair College – IV Sedation and Advanced Cardiac Life Support
- Anesthesia Permit to provide IV Sedation from the State of Ohio
- The Dawson Academy for Advanced Dental Education
- The Las Vegas Institute for Advanced Dental Studies
- The Midwest Implant Institute
- The Misch International Implant Institute
- Many other local and national continuing education programs

Memberships:

- American Dental Society of Anesthesiology
- American Academy of Cosmetic Dentistry
- American Academy of Implant Dentistry
- International College of Oral Implantologists
- Academy of General Dentistry
- American Dental Association
- Ohio Dental Association, Akron Dental Society

Accomplishments:

Putting himself through Case Western University's dental school by working nights at Lawson's bakery and weekends at the Cleveland Clinic, Dr. Marcius opened his first practice at just 24-years-old. After earning a fellowship with the Academy of General Dentistry, he later received his license in IV Sedation—now one of the only dentists in northeast Ohio who provides this service. Dr. Marcius has since completed numerous courses in advanced dentistry to help treat patients with high-anxiety and other forms of compromised health.

Personal:

Dr. Marcius was born in Akron, Ohio, attended St. Vincent High School (now St. V-M) and later the University of Akron. After graduating from Case Western Reserve University School of Dentistry, he opened his first office in Akron's North Hill. Dr. Marcius continues to practice in the Akron area but also enjoys his time off, which he spends with his daughter Chelsia and dog Atticus.

Contact Us:

Joseph G. Marcius, DDS
Chapel Hill Dental Care

1690 Brittain Road
Akron, Ohio 44310
Office: 330-633-711
Fax: 330-633-8837
DrJoeMarcius@earthlink.net